BREATHE WITH ME

Affirmations to Restore Calm,
Heal the Heart and Return to Love

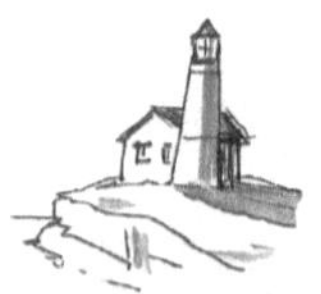

Winter Island Press
Salem, Massachusetts
www.winterislandpress.com

ISBN: 979-8-9925945-8-4
LCCN: 2026909952

Breathe With Me

Affirmations to Restore Calm, Heal the Heart and Return to Love

Karena Virginia

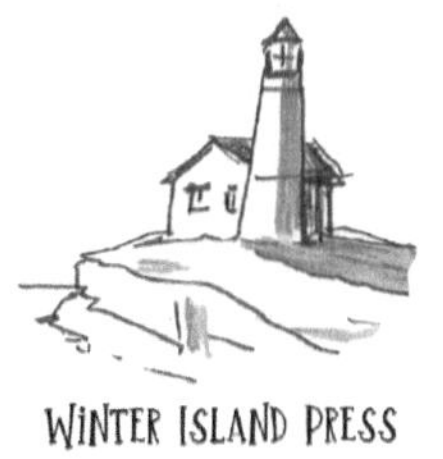

*This is for you, Gabriella and Christian. I love you both more than words can describe. I love you with each breath. I love you with every cell of my body, heart and soul in each moment of existence.
I love you. I love you. I love you.*

Introduction

Blessings to each of you. From my heart to yours, I truly believe that you are holding this book because you are ready to heal. I believe in divine timing, and I believe in miracles.

Welcome back to the comfort and coziness your soul remembers. Welcome home.

◇◇◇

As stories and messages come at us from every direction, many of us are noticing something we may never have imagined in our lifetimes. There is a growing and painful division in our world.

Some of us are opening up, becoming more aware, more flexible…quietly questioning what we once thought we knew and exploring more deeply. We are learning how to bend without breaking, and we are paving the way for stronger, richer resources within ourselves and in the world around us. We are finding our voices and remembering that we matter too, and we are more than enough just as we are.

At the same time, many of us are noticing, with a mix of surprise and unease, that the systems and structures we once thought were steady are shifting before our eyes.

Our minds, bodies and nervous systems are craving an invitation to pause, to breathe, and to discover the inner strength and calm that we know inherently will guide us through uncertain times.

In these pages, you will find gentle affirmations designed to guide you back to your own heart, especially during times of fear, uncertainty, or overwhelm. This book is for anyone who has experienced trauma, for those whose nervous systems need a loving pause, and for anyone seeking comfort in a chaotic world.

Each affirmation is a small beacon of light, a reminder that you are never alone. This is a spiritual book at its heart, honoring the presence of a higher power who loves you unconditionally and is always with you.

You can use this book as a daily messenger. When you need guidance, simply ask, "What is my message for today?" Let your hands open to any page, and trust that the words you land on are the ones meant for you.

Read the affirmation three times while continuing to breathe deeply. You can silently repeat the affirmation throughout the day, especially when you feel triggered or anxious, or you need to shift from a fearful thought to a more loving thought.

Some may keep this book by their bedside as a daily reminder that gentleness, love, comfort and safety are available, and that there are always new choices we can make in life.

With each affirmation, may you feel held, safe, valuable, cared for, comforted, peaceful and cherished. My wish for you is that you remember how very loved you are by affirming the words in this book to your heart with gentleness, inner love and kindness.

We are together on this journey. May angels guide us every step of the way.

With love always.

"You can't stop a fire by running away from it and,
as Karena Virginia's brave words show in her writings,
you can't advance the truth unless you tell it."

Gloria Steinem

"Life is too short for only pink."

I have always loved the color pink. I am all about my light pink pajamas and furry slippers. My first bicycle was pink, and my bedroom was light pink with bright pink and white plaid flowers. My favorite show was Little House; my favorite candy was Brach's pink mints. I even faked being sick when I was little to try Pepto Bismol (only did that once for obvious reasons). Oh, boy.

When my nephew and his cousin passed away within a few months of each other, my heart hurt badly. So much sadness.

But then I realized, we are all in pain. Why is the market for self-help books exploding? We are all searching for a way out of the discomfort.

The other day, I wore a dress and rode a red bicycle around New York City. I felt so free from the sorrow, and a lady yelled at me for being crazy – so I smiled at her. Maybe I was a bit crazy, but my mantra became, "Life is too short for pink, Karena."

I want to be fearless. We have so much work to do as light leaders at this time. We need to be supporting each other and lifting one another up. Life is not about "me," it is about "we," and we are in this together. We are asked to start "we-ing" instead of "me-ing."

I decided to give my niece my pink furry pajamas. I have decided to be brave.

Please join me: What is there to fear except fear itself? I do not want to hide anymore.

Thank you for holding my hand. I will hold yours too.

02

"I live in a world full of miracles."

Do you know that this pressure cooker period you are experiencing is a prep period for the amazing things that are on the way?

The essential ingredient in this thing we call life is to activate the power within us. We all have deep desires that are rooted and sleeping within us. When we awaken them we feel a sense of purpose and magic. However, when we repress them, we feel locked up and stuck. If we do not do the work of unleashing this intense calling, we feel frustrated, angry and trapped.

It's true, we are being shaken up a bit. We are being pressurized like a piece of coal wanting to be a diamond. And just like that piece of coal, we already have everything we need to shine into that brilliance! It is part of our essential nature.

Are you feeling it? Can you recognize that what is ahead is miraculous? Can you breathe through this time of intense transformation? Can you break free of the trap and trust there is a purpose for your unique self? Can you stand up, speak up, and do it?

Let's do this together:

"I live in a world full of miracles."

Shall we?

03

"I believe in me."

We are so divine, so graceful, and so angelic. But we need to be humbly confident in ourselves, or the work of the Divine becomes scattered. We become ineffective until we grasp the reality that God is working through us and breathing into us with every moment. Everything becomes a possibility when we trust the Divine and depend on our own intuitions.

It's hard to feel insecure if we step back and see the big picture. Each breath is a miracle, and our lives are guided by the angels. Self-confidence takes work. It takes fertile environments and self-care. It takes light and self-love. But then, we can build our own self-confidence to trust in a divine plan, trust in the grace of that plan and then, with that trust, everything is possible.

We become love. We become radiant vessels of goodness. We are humbled by our self-confidence. When people operate from their ego, they are coming from a space of insecurity. Our grace is in the self-confidence that we are enough, we are blessed, and we are making the world a better place by sharing our heart.

This is a miraculous mantra:

"I believe in me."

"When I am good, everything around me is good."

Ah! Isn't this the truth? I love when I learn from my clients. This miracle mantra is in honor of a very beautiful woman. She said to me,

"Karena, when I am good, everything around me is good."

YES!

Miracles happen all the time. However, we often block them from occurring in our own lives! We get in our own way. We even resist them at times because of our fears: Fear of failure. Fear of success. Fear of change.

The Divine loves you. Would the Divine give you a miracle if the Divine wasn't going to support you with it? Do you know how much abundance is waiting to enter your life? Or are you thinking in terms of scarcity? This is a big question to work with today, because if you truly knew the way the universe embraces you and holds you, there would never be fear of failure or fear of success. There would be FLOW.

Ever notice when you do your inner work and you uplift your frequency, that everything moves with synchronicity and rhythm?

What do you need to release so you can allow the miracles to enter your life, so you can truly receive?

Let it go.

Trust.

Say this one with me, and change that limited mindset:

"When I am good, everything around me is good."

05

> "Angels are always above me. I am loved,
> supported, and protected at all times."

Whenever I have a particularly challenging week, it is my faith that helps me continue moving forward, sharing what I know to be true. For example: Heaven is real. Angels are guiding us now and always. Just think, maybe the stars in the sky are small openings of light that are shining forth love from our guardian angels. Something I know for sure is that when we lose a loved one, we gain a guardian. Have you ever experienced angels? Have you felt a loved one come through to you from Heaven's gate?

The pain of loss is an earthly discomfort. Loss is an illusion. I have discovered that we never really lose anyone or anything. We do, however, gain more and more love daily. Angels are smiling upon you now. Ask them for their guidance and they will give you a sign. They never disappoint. They always come through. I can feel my nephew as an angel. I see his large smile and I feel his laughter in my heart. His wings have expanded and now he is flying. This one is for you, Michael.

"I forgive myself and grow from my mistakes. Today is a new day."

Every day is a rebirth, a fresh start, and an opportunity to wake up to what is truly important. As we know, our thoughts have a major impact on our day-to-day lives. Using affirmations is a great way to purposefully choose your thoughts and guard against unwanted, negative thoughts. The negative thoughts are really just old chatter, and they are there to remind us to change the channel of our thinking. Many people are feeling a sense of shame, guilt, and exposure at this time.

I notice in my work that we often feel the same emotions collectively. One of the reasons why I am so passionate about mentoring others is because it helps me see how similar we all are. It does not matter if we are famous and in the public eye or if we are private and shy. We are all feeling similar things. We are so much more similar than we recognize.

This truly is a time to rebirth, wake up, start new, attract fresh opportunities, and be kind to ourselves. Life is happening now. Today. Let go of the past, and when the mind fears the future, take a deep breath in and remind your mind that you are so much bigger than those old, stuck, chattering thoughts. Junk that funk! You deserve it.

07

"I'll move that mountain for you."

This miracle mantra came to me while I was riding a bike through a small beach town with my sister. It was my niece's bicycle, which was way too small for me. But I felt happy and free.

That was not an easy summer for my family, as we are all very close, and my nephew passed away that spring. It was our first time at the summer beach house that he was not with us. We were all full of emotions, but there was this beautiful tapestry of love and faith that seemed to carry us forward. As I was riding and hitting my knees into the handlebars, I kept hearing a voice singing in a whisper:

"I'll move that mountain for you."

The breeze reminded me of the gentle touch of angels' wings, and we saw two butterflies on our ride. I knew in my heart that Michael was by our side and the challenges we were experiencing were being comforted by his love. I knew this with every cell in my body. And I realize that it is truly the same for all of you. Miracles are all around you. Healing of mind, body and soul is possible.

Nothing – I repeat, nothing – is impossible.

Can you allow Source energy to move the mountain for you?

08

"I am never upset for the reason I think."

I am constantly amazed at how many miracles occur in our lives when we find a safe place to become vulnerable with one another. It is a very complicated time in the world. We are full of new emotions. We are looking for a guidebook for this time. Yet, there has never been a time like this before. If you are feeling intense feelings of confusion and fear, or if your life is in a huge transition, or you are healing physically, emotionally and/or spiritually, you are among many.

"I am never upset for the reason I think." We may resist this one, because we convince ourselves that we are. But, when we say it to ourselves silently throughout the day, it becomes clear that we are often projecting the past into the present. Asking ourselves when, where, and with whom we have felt the disappointment before, helps us to recognize what we need to heal from our past. Breathe deeply and allow yourself to let the past go. Forgive, release, and heal. You deserve to live a life full of harmony. It is your birthright.

09

"Happiness is within me.
I am embracing happiness now."

Happiness is not something that needs to be achieved. It is an emotion that is within us, and it is calling us to allow it to expand around us. It is a process of lighting ourselves from within while opening our hearts and leaning into our spirit – for this leaning is the key to happiness.

Searching outside of our soul for happiness is not sustainable. Happiness is now. Happiness is in the present moment. Happiness is within.

However, we often have blocks or resistances. We have self-limiting beliefs that clog the pipeline of joy. Our work is to clear them. Eliminate the clutter. The congestion is an energy.

Sometimes we do not know why we feel sad. We may have talked about the same story one hundred times. Visited therapists. Cried to friends. Thought the story was gone, and then – BAM! – it's back.

Ugh.

This is because the story becomes an imprint of ENERGY.

The only way to truly eliminate the pain is by allowing the energy to move. It is ALL in the breath and the space we choose to allow our heart to live in.

Practice this with me:

Rather than working towards happiness, simply let go. Rather than figuring out why things are the way they are, breathe. Rather than numbing the pain, feel it. Then let it lift. Feel it. Then exhale it out. Do this outside. Find a tree, a beach or a garden of flowers. Let nature be your medicine.

And remind yourself of this cosmic law:

"Happiness is within me. I am embracing happiness now."

10

"I place my life in the hands of the Divine. I trust
that the Divine whispers guidance
when I need it most."

Our miracle mantra this week is about trusting that our higher selves are being guided by divine energy at all times, and we can always choose to go with the flow. We can let go without giving in. We can surrender our concerns and listen to the guidance that speaks to us in our heart, this gentle and sweet area of our being. This is where the Divine whispers which way to step and reminds us when it is time to find silence and let go of our oars so the mystical ocean can take us to our highest calling and destination.

Today, let's take time to trust the flow, recognizing that challenges arrive when we are being guided to close a door and open another one. Actually, when we flow and listen, the door opens on its own.

"I embrace my value, no matter what anyone else says or thinks."

This miracle mantra is the result of ten quiet and contemplative days in Italy. It is usually when we are unplugged from technology that we feel the most connected to Source.

While we were walking through a small village on the outskirts of Venice, I saw a painting on the wall of an old building. I was mesmerized by it. There wasn't anyone else around but my family and me, so there was not any hype around it. (Usually when there is a line to see something, it is human nature to think it must be special.) However, this painting was simply under layers of old paint. While taking it in, I realized that it must have been painted during Renaissance period, then painted over as were so many miraculous pieces of art in Italy at that time. Did this artist recognize his/her gift? Or did he/she feel it was not good enough?

Thinking about this brought me to consider my own life. How often I question how comfortable I feel sharing my gifts. What if I am misunderstood? What if I succeed so much, others do not want to be around me anymore? What if my sharing steps on another's toes? Or, what if it offends someone?

Well, none of this is actually our business. If we follow the guidance system in our hearts, we must be bold and courageous. We must trust that we are protected when we share our gifts with the world. We were made to do this!

Do you ever feel afraid of shining? Think on this, for a moment.

It does not matter what anyone else thinks if you are living from your heart. And you can't change anyone else, either. However, you can recognize that it is safe to expose your gifts. Otherwise, your unique purpose remains hidden. And we ALL have unique and valuable gifts. When we share what we have been brought here to share, we are serving the highest good. If our 'gift' gets painted over, it's not our problem anymore! We did our work.

I urge you all to shine!

12

"There goes my brain, doing that thing
it does again."

We cannot deny that the world is moving faster than we can keep up with. There is so much information, stimulation, and constancy. When I was in my twenties, I lived in New York City (the city that never sleeps), and now I live outside of the hustle and bustle. However, life is moving faster than ever. The city that never sleeps was less crazy than the parks are today. Everything keeps going. Remember when we were younger, and a snow day meant a day off? Now a day without meetings is a day to catch up on emails. We are all in this together, and that means we can remind one another that we are enough without constantly doing.

A dear friend of mine gave me this quote, and I have been using it all week long. Whenever my mind gets over-stimulated or fearful, I stop and repeat this to myself. Then I take a moment to remember that there is a divine plan at play. Certain things are out of my control, but I am not a static being. I am a being that vibrates constantly, and my thoughts are being directed out into the universe. It is the same for you. We are energy. If our energy is of love, we will attract more love. If our thoughts are loving, we vibrate that same frequency and become magnetic beings attracting more of it.

When the mind gets wonky this week, take a deep breath in

and remember that you are so much more than your mind games. Then silently repeat this affirmation:

"There goes my brain doing that thing it does again."

Trust me. It works.

13

"I am open to miracles in my life."

This miracle mantra seems obvious, but it was a long time coming.

As many of you know, my nephew passed away some time ago. While the first week was spent in shock and spending every second with my family, the next week was putting the pieces back together, and the week after that was using everything I had to lift my mother and my brother into a sense of hope. It wasn't until after all that, that I realized my nervous system felt shaky, and my body was tired.

Yet despite all this, the message is that miracles are real. I also know that Heaven is the most beautiful existence, and angels surround us at all times. The hardest part of losing a loved one is the struggle of sorrow that exists on the earth realm.

Shortly after Michael's death, I also spent time in Colorado with my incredible publishing team at Sounds True. The team working with me was a pure miracle. I was able to compartmentalize my feelings of loss, and I was able to pose for pictures for four days straight. I even laughed – true heartfelt laughs of joy. Everything about the photo shoot was pure bliss. Every person at Sounds True touched my heart. It was as if a miracle was being created with all our hearts merging into the art. And in the ethers there was an angel, Michael. He is our living angel. While he will be forever missed, his light will shine upon so many teens who are feeling the pain of the world.

My prayer is that these miracle mantras and my love for all of you shines on the world in the same way. I do love deeply. I am certain it is part of the divine plan. Please use this miracle mantra as we allow the miracles to flow upwards, inwards, around us and towards those we love:

"I am open to miracles in my life."

14

"I am taking time for self-care."

We need self-care right now more than ever before. Sometimes I fantasize about living in the olden days, with beautiful fireplaces and the scent of homemade pies and hearty soup on the hearth. Quiet evenings with a candle and a book. I know this is me being all romantic, because life was not easy in those days either. However, do you ever crave a day where you can unplug from electronics? Do we realize what we are doing to our nervous systems by texting, emailing, social media-ing, snap chatting, and then obsessing about what we've texted, emailed, social media-ed, snap chatted, and spent yesterday obsessing over? Yep. This is what our lives have become. So!

We have to make a choice. A simple choice to take time every day to care for our heart and soul. That may mean setting boundaries with our phones, or it may mean leaving our phones in the car the next time we stroll through the supermarket. It may be something like spending a few minutes meditating each morning, before checking your phone. You know what you need. Can you treat yourself to the gift of self-care? Start with the affirmation, and watch how your mind listens.

"I am taking time for self-care."

15

"Who Am I?"

Self-inquiry is indispensable to the journey of our spirit. When we peer deeply into the vastness of our own being, we also look into the infinite depths of the universe. Self-inquiry is not about arriving at a definition. It is about peeling away the layers, deepening into clarity and realization throughout our lives, and understanding that no matter what happens on the journey, we are the observer, the pure "me" that is watching our own mind.

Maharishi Mahesh Yogi, one of the first Indian spiritual teachers who brought Transcendental Meditational to thousands in the West, used to say that in order to free ourselves from doubt and fear, we sincerely must ask ourselves, "Who am I?" This self-investigation is essential to our development. And it never ends. Maharishi explained that no wisdom outside of ourselves will ever help us the same way that we can help ourselves.

A miracle is a healing that occurs when we surrender the outcome. After many years of wanting to fit in and hiding my deep spiritual connection to the unseen world, I have finally entered the place where I can say, "I am me and that is enough." For example, the other day a friend and I were talking, and I felt very misunderstood by a comment she made. In the past, I may have jumped to defending myself. On this day, however, I took a deep breath and found myself at peace with her perception being very different than mine; I could recognize the beauty in both our points of view. There was a deeper level of acceptance, and at that deeper level, no need for reaction. I consider moments like this to be miracles.

We can go deep within ourselves and recognize that with our strengths, weaknesses, fears, successes, doubts, esteems, and adequacies or inadequacies, we are ourselves – and that is perfect. If we answer the question with truth, we can say: "Me! I am me. I am here experiencing this life, and my intuition is the vehicle that guides me. I am home."

You are home! And your home is beautiful. No one can take your home away, and you can decorate your home however you'd like. Now, that is freeing. Isn't it time you love yourself for who you are? Take a deep seat inside your soul, and listen to the mystery as it sings in perfect harmony. You can say this mantra throughout the day. Let it do its work. It doesn't take much, but it heals much.

"Who am I?"

16

"The triggers are liberating me."

We all carry baggage from our past, like an old, heavy suitcase full of limiting beliefs that we drag around with us wherever we go. And when someone starts to go through our bag, we feel triggered. However, our awareness of these triggers is the very thing that can liberate us from holding so tightly to the attachments that hold us back from shining!

I used to hide my light so that others could shine. It made me feel like I would be accepted and welcomed if I sat quietly and let them have the power. After years of allowing this sort of behavior, I finally hit rock bottom when someone I trusted pulled the carpet from under me. I looked up to her. I revered her spiritually as well as emotionally. It hurt so darn much. But I allowed it. I even attracted it.

It turned out to be the greatest gift. It forced me to reclaim my shine. I would not be meeting with TV networks now, if I was still hiding. I urge you to reclaim your brilliance too. All these triggers are simply gifts to help you drop the heavy bag. Let it go. Let it go!

17

"I find deep peace in living my truth."

I am hoping you will find this mantra at exactly the right time. Like all these affirmations, it is designed to shift our limiting beliefs from doubt to faith.

We learn to question ourselves from a very young age, and our work throughout life is often a journey of erasing shame while loving ourselves exactly as we are. If something needs to change for the highest good, we can pray for the change. Beating ourselves up is counterproductive. Allowing the shift to occur naturally from prayer is the miracle that we can create through thoughts, energy, and self-compassion. Guilt is not helpful. Fear is stifling. Finding peace in the midst of chaos is a much kinder way to be with ourselves.

Start with a deep breath and the miracle mantra:

"I find deep peace in living my truth."

18

"I am happy. I am me. I am enough."

Life is a playground when we stop expecting to be hurt. Remember when we were younger – we'd fall and get back up, and then we'd fall again, and get back up! We learned to ride a bicycle and balance on the monkey bars, and we didn't mind falling in the process. As adults, we often forget that we have a support system of angels that hold us. If we fall, we will get back up with their assistance. Sometimes we are called to have fun and take a little chance. If we let our fear of playing big take over, we miss the chance to touch others the way our souls are meant to.

Remember the first day of school? That fear of inhabiting a space larger than what we were used to? Then on our last day of school, it seemed so small! We were then entering an entirely new space of college or work that seemed too big for us, again. But that is all an illusion, because nothing is too big for our soul – except for fear itself.

This miracle mantra is to release the fear that holds us back from being the light we are meant to be. Spirit is on our side when we lead with the heart.

Allowing our radiance to shine gives others the opportunity to do the same. We can take a chance. We can be silly. We can be less than perfect without feeling shame. We can be our individual selves and recognize that we are more than enough.

"I look up and I can feel a touch of grace."

It is not an easy time. I know this to be true for many of us. Sometimes I feel as though I am lost in the mess of my mind. I do not pretend to have all the answers, because I do not believe any of us in the earth realm do.

I do not understand spiritual manipulation at all!

Spirituality is love. All acceptance. Oneness.

We can write books on spirituality, but if we do not walk our talk, how can we sell them consciously? And today I feel this so deeply – I need to look up. What is going on in the world of spirituality?

It is time to be real. It is time to find our own personal truths. Maybe there is something triggering you somewhere in your own life. Those emotions are real.

LOOK UP.

It is the only way to rise above the things that do not work for us. Upwards, there is perfection. When I look up, bliss overflows from my heart, and all the chaos and confusion of my mind disappears. When I look up, I see miracles.

20

"Everything I am searching for
is already within me."

Life is moving fast. Our days are filled with emails, texts, schedules, and rushing from one thing to the next. It is so easy to feel less-than when we compare ourselves to others. Comparison has become an epidemic now that technology is so accessible. Then there is that ugly word, jealousy. The emotion that creates an urge to find something outside of ourselves in order to numb our feelings of inadequacy. I have seen even the most spiritual people I know get caught in the jealousy trap. It is a primal emotion.

How do we get out of the sticky trap?

Every time you feel triggered, rushed, less-than, disempowered, or fearful, see it as a chance to put this into practice:

1. Breathe deeply.
2. Laugh (even if you need to force it).
3. Tap your index finger to the center of your forehead for a minute.
4. Silently say, "Everything I am searching for is already within me."
5. Drink a tall glass of water.

And if you are able to go outside, take a walk. Observe how nature never pushes, rushes, or compares. Nature simply is.

And nature works quite efficiently. The acorn becomes the tree. The seed the flower. The sun rises without question.

We are no different than nature, but we have a nervous system and a mind that keeps us caught in the illusion that we must search, rush, and strive. But none of this is necessary. Your radiance, projection, and presence are more than enough.

"I lovingly embrace all my emotions with compassion."

Something in the world is shifting in a big way. People are experiencing feelings that may have been repressed or may have never been explored, but now they are surfacing. Many people are crying as part of the cleansing process. These tears bring relief from the emptiness and longing.

But what is the longing? What is happening? Wherever we are, we feel we are supposed to be somewhere else. But what is on the other side? It is all an illusion.

We are meant to be exactly where we are right now. The tears are actually beautiful expression of love, because our hearts are opening and loving beyond our normal capacity. The tears are flushing away our frustrations and enabling us to love beyond limitations. Beneath the hurt, we are experiencing an odd sense of peace. This is a calling at this time, an energetic request from all creation. Let the sadness go with the tears and free yourself from the confusion. Allow yourself to laugh and cry at the same time.

Allow it.

Free yourself.

Find the pause between the tears and embrace the stillness. You are not going crazy. You are simply allowing yourself to feel and expand in ways you may have never known you could. You are not alone, so remember this, as well: when we share our vulnerability, we give others permission to do the same.

22

"Ask. Yes. Believe. Yes. Receive. Yes."

You have read about it, heard about it, and contemplated it, but do you practice it? Do you believe it?

We are co-creators.

Source energy is always matching our belief system based on our thoughts. What are you thinking today?

Say this affirmation with me, and believe the words you are saying – for you have more power than you know.

"Ask. Yes. Believe. Yes. Receive. Yes. Thank you."

23

"My true strength comes from within."

Sometimes, we go through periods where everything hurts. We feel so raw, even old hurts from the past start resurfacing. Can this be a gift? It may not feel like one, but challenges often bring opportunities. Even the hurts can strengthen us. The next time you hurt, feel it. Where does it hurt? Release it. You have to feel it to heal it. If you try to ignore it, you are simply hoarding it, and the more we hoard, the more we repress.

The truth is, we will never find a sustainable source of comfort outside of us. We can find temporary fixes, but true strength comes from within. Ever feel like a branch blowing in the wind? The solution is within you. When those moments appear, close your eyes, pucker your lips and inhale like you are drawing in air through a straw. Hold the air in and let it give you strength. Exhale and release whatever is disappointing you. Give it to the wind. Release the hurt. Let the wind take your concern, but use your strength to ground yourself and silently repeat this mantra:

"My true strength comes from within."

24

"Unity connects us to the light."

We are devastated by war and acts of violence, and it is easy to become weighed down with sadness. It's too much for us to cope with, on our own; there is too much to fear and too much weight to carry around. We do not understand why such awful tragedies hurt such innocent souls. It seems so unfair. Yet, we have two choices. We can freeze in sadness and fear, or we can connect with the light in love.

We can't make sense of tragedy in this dimension, but the heavens show us that love and light prevail. We must transcend our physical fears and connect to the higher realm where love, purity, and perfection reside. Heaven is real. Heaven is love.

Uniting in prayer activates the light. If we can pray deeply together, we can manifest that light and help it shine throughout our world. We are small, but together we are gigantic.

Today, pray for peace. Please share this mantra, and hold hands with one another and unite in the light.

25

"I am worthy of giving and receiving love."

This mantra reminds me of Rumi's poem:

When Love comes suddenly and taps
on your window, run and let it in,
but first shut the door of your reason,
even the smallest hint chases love away …

If we just share our hearts, things will be better. We can't expect the love to be returned by the same person, but we are guaranteed to receive love in return. This is the law of quantum physics!

I have a very open heart; I have been open and loving my entire life. It's the Italian in me! Sometimes I open my heart so much because it is natural for me, and while it is not always reciprocated by the person it is going to at the moment, it is still always returned.

The key is to trust that love is energy.

What we give, we receive. It is a spiritual law as well.

Also, we have to allow the love back in! Receiving love can be surprisingly difficult. We do not know how worthy we are of being loved; if we did our world would be one big heart full of peace.

This mantra is a reminder of the importance of our connections to people. Don't judge what your heart tells you. Listen to the lovely voice of your soul. You do not have to prove anything. Just open a little deeper and trust what you find. Remember, when we open our hearts wider to receive the love that the universe pours into us, we are healing ourselves. Please join me this week as we focus and vibrate our miracle mantra:

"I am worthy of giving and receiving love."

"I am sorry. I love you. Please forgive me. I thank you."

Ho'oponopono is a Hawaiian healing practice which means to clear obstacles and make things right. By feeling and saying the words, "I'm sorry, I love you, please forgive me, I thank you," we take responsibility for ourselves and the world we create. It is said that this affirmation can attract miracles.

So many of our core challenges come from the old stories we store in our minds and energy fields. In the Hawaiian culture, there is a belief that what we say and do will affect future generations, and what we feel now is a result of the generations before us. This resonates with me so much as I am realizing more and more that the blocks we experience are not solely in our mind. They are also imprinted in our DNA.

Affirmations can truly shift us into clearer versions of our inner beauties by assisting us in moving beyond the resistances of mind, energy, and physiology.

I love how I feel saying this prayer. It is such a gift to learn from others, and I feel very grateful to you for allowing me to be a vessel that can share from my heart. I truly feel happiness from giving.

"I am sorry. I love you. Please forgive me. I thank you."

"The purity of my heart stands by me."
˜ Yogi Ji

This miracle mantra is universal. The love, purity, compassion, and kindness we give to others are enough to sustain us in all our endeavors. This is the law of quantum physics and spirituality. It is where science and the Divine meet. What we put out always comes back. Like attracts like. When we give, we receive.

Today is a day to let go of expectations and remember what is truly important. Love. It is better to feel good than to feel right. Choosing love for ourselves and others becomes a magical cycle of endless play when we surrender our expectations. We can only do this sincerely when we trust that the higher realms are watching. I believe we reap what we sow, but sometimes it takes seasons. What we sow in one season, we may not reap until the next. Sometimes we are tested with patience. Breath can help. Place your hand on your heart and remember:

"The purity of my heart stands by me."

28

"I recognize that God is with me. Always."

I have recently learned to accept, I cannot be anyone but me. While I have beautiful friends in the entertainment industry and friends who are 'famous,' all that truly matters is how I feel when I am with them. Sometimes I feel alone in 'conscious' environments, while I feel very welcome on Broadway in New York City.

I have learned something in a profound and challenging way. I have learned to look beyond illusions and to see what is real. What is real is LOVE, and love arrives when we allow it in. Love cannot be controlled, and we hurt our own souls when we think that love is available only in 'certain environments.'

God is with us everywhere.

Let's stop assuming we need to be someone we are not.

Just BE YOU. And remember:

God is with you, ALWAYS. And everywhere.

29

"I will help you."

Today, it is time to slow down, reflect, forgive, heal and open to the wonders of the Divine. Sometimes, we forget how to do this!

When I was writing this mantra, the word that kept showing up for me to write about was 'forgiveness.' What do you need to forgive in order to free yourself from hurt?

Forgiveness is not an easy thing to do. It is actually one of the hardest things for human beings to do. But anger is poison in your body. And you deserve to free yourself from that poison.

Closing your eyes, connecting to the everlasting love of God, and asking for strength, support, and guidance can be your miracle. It can purify you.

Imagine this miracle mantra as if it is a whisper from the Divine, and as you repeat it over and over, feel as if the words are coming from the angels. Feel as if the words are soft and nurturing, like a warm, cozy blanket on a cold day. Listen to the angels as they sing:

"I will help you."

"I release all self-limiting stories about myself."

We were born knowing our needs would be met. We did not have to desire it, we knew as infants that when we cried, we would be taken care of. How do we know this is true? Because, if it were not true, in at least a basic sense, we would not be here today. We were fed and cared for, yet at a very early age we still learned to believe the self-limiting stories that we tell ourselves as adults.

We did not need to understand language; it was in the look and feel of our caregivers. We don't remember (in our conscious minds) the moments when we were most vulnerable, yet our energy fields hold these moments as if they are tangible pieces of evidence that we are not worthy of love.

Let's be honest. We all have those moments, and we all hold self-limiting stories in our energetic body, our subconscious minds, and even our conscious minds, unless (until!) we do our work to clear them.

Please remember that it is okay to crave personal freedom from the chains of false beliefs. Many of these beliefs were not our own in the first place, yet we got caught up in believing we were not lovable unless we were living up to the ideals of others.

Free yourself. See it. Feel it. And then LET IT GO. Allow yourself to reconnect to your earliest self, the time when love was the only emotion you felt, understood, and knew. You are loved for being you. You are perfect just the way you are.

31

"God's Love sustains me."

This is a great, simple truth. We all have different background, but we all have access to Grace, Gratitude, and God. God sustains us, always.

May God bless you.

32

"My life is in harmony with my truth."

This mantra offers a profound opportunity for release and healing. It is an invitation to align our outer self-expression with our innermost concept of who we are. By saying this mantra, a gateway is opened through which we may move past any outer circumstances that are not in alignment with the beautiful depths of our inner beings, and press up into the light of true expression. It is a time for shedding what confines us. It is time to grow like flowers emerging from the soil.

As we grow, we may have a little soil on our new leaves, but it quickly falls away. When we move past what no longer serves us, we can walk forward with gratitude, without that weight, growing into light, walking with love, through new pathways that have been waiting for us. Let us align our outer harmony in a way that reflects the true depths of what we feel inside. May this miracle mantra help you move into renewal and growth.

"I easily release the old and happily embrace the new."

This is a mantra for self-renewal and taking extra care of ourselves and our health. When we love ourselves, we generate a powerful frequency which attracts our spiritual counterparts so we can co-create and shine. Radiance is created naturally by the ability to love ourselves deeply enough that we can love others. Then we shine love and light out from the fullness of our hearts.

As we renew our intention to live as beings of love, it helps to cleanse our physical body, as well. Eat light, healthy food and breathe deep, cleansing breaths. Do a liver detox to remove old toxins. Cold showers in the morning will help with circulation and get your skin glowing. Get a massage if you can. Take time for a yoga class, and go for a walk outside in fresh air. Sending you love, light, and radiance.

"I am safe and sound. All is well."

There is so much happening in the world right now, do you feel the heightened energy? At times like these, our insecurities can be triggered, communication can be confusing, and lessons can keep showing up. But we have a choice. We can ride the wave and accelerate alongside the energy that attracts our deepest hearts' desires, or we can get stuck in the web of fear. Whatever is taking place for you, remember fear is an illusion. Whenever you feel scattered, just affirm the truth and shift into the frequency of LOVE. You are not alone in this huge transformation!

Anything is possible–now more than ever! Clear your mind, open your heart and focus your attention on what you most desire. It is time to align with the infinite, brilliant, unlimited possibility that is your highest spiritual light and authentic truth. I repeat: the time is now more than ever.

Let's manifest brilliance together!

"Give it all up, and get it all back."

This miracle affirmation came to me while my husband and
I were sitting under the most beautiful fragrant flowers at
Hacienda Siesta Alegre. The birds were singing, and the scents
of flowers and fire were blending into an old world fragrance
that our souls seemed to remember.

I was thinking about the way our minds operate with attachment. It is the reptilian brain that holds and grasps, and we all
have it. Even the most enlightened beings on Earth have the
challenges of 'mine.'

This is not something to be ashamed of, it is something to
be aware of, so we can work through the ego and enter the
heart. It is an ongoing practice.

The reptilian brain tricks us, but once we recognize this trick-
ster is at play, we can take charge and listen to our heart. This
is where true beauty happens. When we let go of something,
it comes back if it is meant to, or we discover we were better
off without it. But often something even better replaces it.

As the full moon eclipse is on its way, see if you can meditate
on this thought: what we are not willing to give up becomes
a fear. Love exalts us. Letting go is actually about trusting the
principals of life that are way bigger than the mind.

36

"Love is in me and around me."

It is easy to forget the Love that surrounds us, fills us, and embraces us all the time. It is a frequency that lives to our left and to our right, and deeply within our hearts. It is a vibration of sound that our ears often do not hear, even as it resounds above, below, and within the center of our being every moment of every day.

Why do we get caught up in fear instead of love? Why do we question ourselves and feel emotions that tangle us up instead of giving us peace? Because we are spiritual beings learning, evolving and growing. True self-esteem requires application. Life experiences get caught in the very structure of our beings, and if we do not remind ourselves of the beauty around us, we can get caught in the trap of fear.

Let's do this work together. We all need this reminder. I will meet you in the field of all possibilities as we meditate with this miracle mantra:

"Love is in me and around me."

You are loved—deeply, unequivocally, and unconditionally loved.

"I am aligning with my deepest desires now."

When we find balance, we find health, joy, and a pathway to miracles. Yin and yang, feminine and masculine, sun energy and lunar energy, asleep and awake–there are two sides to all aspects of our lives.

In the neutral space where the opposites are in balance, there is a miraculous passageway to fulfillment. This is the road to the magic of co-creation. From harmony we can attract miracles.

Remember, affirmations work on our energy field through repetition. Say this mantra aloud for three minutes a day to enhance your intentions in very profound ways.

38

"Time is a gift. I choose to love."

Life gets so busy. Sometimes we go-go-go without pausing for stillness and reflection. But time is the one thing we can never get back.

We can lose love, and it can return; we can lose money, and it can return–yet, when we lose time, it never comes back.

When we make a conscious effort to choose love, we are making the most of our time in this world. Love is always the answer. Love is the highest of all frequencies. Loving will never end. Life is a precious gift that does not last long. I choose to love. Will you join me?

"Love is the light that keeps me safe from fear."

This mantra is a reminder to allow the light of love to illuminate your fears so they can dissolve and dissipate.

I feel fear when I am riding in the passenger seat of a fast-moving car on the highway. I feel even more fear if it's night, or if my children are in the car. The fear is so strong that I can feel my entire body tighten with tension, and after a long car ride I often have a clenched jaw. I practice deep breathing, and I pray, yet something still takes over. I know many of you experience fears like this, as well.

I believe that our DNA is imprinted with past trauma from our ancestral lineage. We are prone to fears that come from the wounds of our ancestors.

My father was in a car accident on a highway at night when he was a teenager, and his father was driving. His father lost control of the car and was killed. It happened fifteen years before I was born, but I feel the trauma in my subconscious.

This mantra reminds me to let light and love melt away the energy of fear. May it remind you, too, and may you see the beauty, the potential, and the wonders of the universe. Fear is an illusion.

"My outer expressions mirror my inner truth."

I think we can all say, we are ready to be true to ourselves!

A beautiful miraculous harmony occurs when our outer expression emulates our inner truth. The universe works in tandem with our thoughts and feelings. We have reached a courageous pivotal time. We are enough, and even with our imperfections and our doubts, we are valuable! All of us.

We are being called to act, love, speak, and walk with truth. Aren't we tired of faking it? We can be freed from worrying about the judgments of others, freed from the impossible task of trying to please everyone, and freed from our own crippling self-judgments, by acting on the knowledge that our inner truth is divinely implanted within our soul. When we do this, everything else falls into alignment, and the doors to miraculous co-creative synergy swing open.

This is the calling of our era.

We have to be real and true to our inner divinity in order to feel free. The fakin' it stuff just ain't makin' it anymore! This I know in my own life, and I urge you to be courageous with me. Does it really matter if we are not accepted for our truth, if we are being true to ourselves? Nope. If we are pleasing others while hiding behind mask, we are giving away our power.

Let's free ourselves and reclaim our power! NOW.

"Whatever you ask for in prayer, believe that you have received it, and it will be yours."

I have spent a lot of time at the beach just watching the water move and the sun rise and set. It gives me the greatest sense of connection to myself. Once when I was watching the tide, I thought, "If we truly trust the Divine, why are we so full of doubt, insecurity, and fear?" The answer came to me in an instant.

We allow our minds to run the show, and our minds are full of illusions. The only true way to move beyond the mind games is to drop into the heart space. The only way to stay in the heart center is through trusting the presence of Spirit.

Have you ever noticed that there are churchgoers who attend worship yet are not open to discussing the heart and prayer? We are conditioned to be shy about using certain words such as God, Love, and Heaven. Yet, these are words of hope and possibility. Showing up in holy places is great. Practicing what holy places represent is key.

I believe in the power of prayer. I believe in it with every cell of my body. I know Heaven is real. I know angels exist. I know you are being cared for with a love that is beyond the mind's capacity for understanding.

Please trust me in this. I would not say this sort of thing if I didn't know it. It's not just a belief. I have seen beyond the veil of this dimension.

Love is truly with you, right NOW!

42

"My inner light sustains me."

Our sensitivity gives us the ability to see beyond the density and anger of the world, yet it also provides us with a powerful awareness of all that is happening. Being aware of the truth in situations can feel quite lonely at times, because seeing hidden agendas feels like knowing a secret that nobody else wants to know! But many of us are feeling this way, these days. We see our friends or loved ones being taken advantage of, or we sense danger in the air, but there is not any factual evidence to support our intuitive knowing.

There is a gift in all of this, though! Once we learn to accept the dualistic nature of human beings, we realize that while people can be disappointing and hurtful, and some people do have selfish motives, our inner light will ALWAYS sustain us.

Smiling and allowing our own love to radiate is the greatest remedy for hurt. If you ever question your intuition, put your thumb and index finger together and create a circle with each hand. Close your eyes. Breathe. With practice, the answers will arrive through your inner guidance system. Trust this. Your inner guidance has all the answers. No matter what comes through, let your inner guidance system be full of light, and project that light out. Nothing is more powerful than rising above.

Today, we state our miracle affirmation with our thumbs and

index fingers touching to create a flowing circle of awareness. Sitting for three minutes and affirming "My inner light sustains me" will enable us to rise above the situations that confuse us. We will gain clarity, and we will free ourselves from any pain the truth brings up for us.

43

> "Out beyond ideas of
> wrongdoing and rightdoing,
> there is a field. I'll meet you there."
> ~ Rumi

I love this poem because it helps me to remember that there is a space where we can meet challenges with neutrality.

Sometimes when I feel frustrated, I stop myself, take a deep breath, and repeat this verse to myself as a mantra.

We can't control the actions of others, but we can control our reactions to their actions. One of the greatest ways to practice peace is to breathe deeply before speaking. When we respond with a kneejerk reaction, we can easily say things we regret. I have an affirmation that I say to myself, and it has helped me in so many ways: "Inhale. Don't react. Exhale."

While I am breathing, I focus on the higher realms so I can see beyond the right and wrong of actions into the fullest potential that lies within each individual when it is invoked. If another person is not ready to activate the light, I can send them my light from a distance. Maybe even meet them in that field of neutrality.

Sending love from my heart to the heavens and then directly to your heart.

44

"I live my life with my inner light guiding me."

I have always been in awe of Renaissance art and cherubs. I often walk through museums or churches in a meditative state of amazement for the miracles that humans have been able to channel.

When we live our lives allowing our hearts to show us our next step, miracles happen. Sometimes we find ourselves talking to a stranger and telling them something they need to hear, but we are just vessels for Grace. When we let our inner light guide us in life, we can just show up and trust the miracle of each moment.

I held a woman last night as she cried in my arms. All I know is that her name is Susan and her husband and father are both in the hospital. Something moved me to walk up to her while she was hiding behind a smile at a restaurant. It was not me. It was Grace.

This miracle mantra is a reminder of the perfect order of our heart's callings:

"I live my life with my inner light guiding me."

Everything is in perfect order. There are miracles everywhere. Sometimes we just need to take a breath and observe them in silence.

45

"I am stepping out of the shadows and into the light."

We are all being guided to grow, and growing can be uncomfortable. Be kind to yourself. Let yourself be YOU. The YOU in YOU is a gift. There is no reason to hide in the shadows. It is time to discern our own shadows and consciously step into what we know is true. Trusting our heart is the only way.

When we allow ourselves to pay attention to our inner world, we can also step free of darkness. We shine light into all the corners, and that light transforms us. Allow yourself to clearly discern. Is a thought bringing you down? Notice the thought very closely. Really observe and analyze it. Determine if it is real or if it is based on a shadow from the past. Notice how it comes and goes. If it is real, is there is a possibility you can also see a glimpse of angelic love shining on the situation? If it is a shadow from the past, can you shine light on it? The only thing that can truly make a shadow disappear is light. Shine that light with your attention.

Breathe in. Exhale. Doesn't that feel better?

"I am stepping out of the shadows and into the light."

<h1 style="text-align:center">46</h1>

"I am growing and expanding and
getting better and better every day."

We all have things to work on. One of my biggest lessons has been to feel free being myself without worrying about what others think. A few years ago, my work was to love myself daily, instead of crying every day for the pain in my heart when my father passed away. We are all in "the school of life," as spiritual souls having human experiences, and sometimes we feel like we are graded for our accomplishments!

This miracle mantra helps us to improve on ourselves without comparing or competing with anyone else. Everyone has their tests. You never know what the person you feel most envious of may be going through privately. Don't compare. And if you must compete, compete with yourself through consistent self-improvement.

"Nothing can dim my light when it shines from within."

I love teaching. I love it so much, because it gives me an opportunity to share in such an authentic way. The ego steps aside and the heart speaks. One of the most beautiful lessons I have learned through teaching is that authenticity is enough. We do not need to prove anything to anyone else. When someone reacts with negativity to the love and light we are sharing in life, we can see that they are just in fear. All actions—even beautiful ones—have reactions. It's science.

When our actions stem from the heart, the reactions of others just don't matter. It's time for us to be courageous and let our truth shine out. If our truth comes from genuine love, even if it threatens someone, they will find a lesson in it. It will help them to grow. This is the law of the universe.

48

"Grace is all around me today."

There are blessings all around you, and many of them are gifts you have not yet noticed. The dreams that have not yet manifested are the dreams that God is working on with you right now. If you look with gratitude at what you have right now, you will uplift your happiness. It is so much easier to focus on what is lacking, yet gratitude for small and simple forms of abundance will create an expansion in the energy of your dreams.

The gifts that we have and the dreams we desire all begin as thoughts, emotions, energy, prayer, and love. And they are here right now. Look at all the good in your life and say, "Wow – thank you." If it seems like you are lacking in some way, find a place of abundance in your life, and focus your energy there. Changing your emotions and creating from a place of empowerment will shift you into a higher frequency. This new frequency has the potential to replace what is missing into what is manifesting.

"Grace is all around me today."

Expect miracles.

49

"I open my heart to life."

When I was a child, I wanted my name to be Alison. My very best friend was Ali, and in my eyes she was perfect. I was so different, and I just wanted to fit in with the pack. The child who is different is often left out.

As an adult, I have embraced my deep and sensitive nature. I used to fear not being invited to the party; however, I have learned that the real party is within my heart. When I open my heart to my authentic truth, I am no longer afraid to stand apart. My truth sets me free to align with my highest aspirations. The key is to do it with unlimited amounts of love for the self and for the world. It is truly alright to walk a path that has not been walked before when we are living with love, integrity, truth, and trust in the gift of individuality.

I used to hear, "She is so weird" when I was a child; yet I now celebrate that cute little weirdo who loves so deeply. She is love. I want you to see that beautiful inner child in yourself, too. Love her. Love him. Know that it is totally okay to be yourself, to love yourself. And once you do, you have created a miracle.

50

"I release the thoughts that hold me back from living the life of my dreams. I am attracting my deepest desires now."

You are so loved. Angels are with you. Get out of your head! The mind is the only obstacle. You have the power to create the life of your dreams. Dream Big. The time is Now. Miracles surround you. Let go. Let God.

51

"I open my heart and let God fill it with love."

Today, let's practice keeping our hearts open. The angels are keeping us safe, and they want us to ask them for their assistance. These are magical times, and miracles are everywhere. We have everything we need to co-create with God, but we must choose Love over fear. If fear or doubt creep in, we must tend the darkness with light and love. If we get stuck, we can take deep breath and fill our lungs with love. Love has the power to transform fear. Love is the substance that miracles depend on. Love is all we need, dear friends.

From my heart to yours, I pray for all of you who are reading this. May we surrender and trust that everything is being organized in Heaven for us here on Earth. Our souls know this truth, yet our minds forget.

Let's remember this together:

"I open my heart and let God fill it with love."

> "I learn from everything I do.
> There are no failures."

We all go through cycles where everything seems wonky. Communication is filled with misunderstandings, and we question what we and others are doing, and why. If we do not work on tuning our thoughts to positivity, our insecurities will always win. Everyone struggles with self-doubt and all sorts of fears. I repeat: EVERYONE!

Those of us who are sensitive will often question ourselves for our actions, worry about how we are perceived and received, and regret stating things that our hearts needed to say. That is okay. Each day is a lesson. If we are self-aware and learn from our mistakes, we will grow into stronger and wiser beings. We can use the gift of affirmation to elevate our thoughts from fear and negativity to hope and positivity.

53

"There is a light all around me that protects,
heals, and nourishes me always."

Creation begins in the magical realm of thoughts. There is an energy field around us and within us, and this is the vibrational origin of all that exists–it is the realm where angels sing. As humans, we can co-create our realities by working with the vibration in this field of prayer.

Despite having this power, we are often limited by our past, our memories, or emotions like guilt and fear, which can leave residual scars, tears, and opacities in our personal energy field. We are sometimes told that all we have to do is change our mind, shift our thoughts, and thereby change our lives, as though this were as simple as flicking a switch. But that philosophy can lead to self-judgment and feelings of failure, as we start to wonder why it is not so easy to keep our thoughts positive. Shifting our thought field is not that simple!

The challenge is to heal and harmonize our long-term memory wounds in order align our mental projections with our soul. Long-term memory wounds are often sensed as triggers for reactions, those things that push our buttons.

Miracles happen when we pray for the healing of our scars and fill our wounds with love, breath, and light, especially through prayer. Saying prayers and mantras out loud can counteract the waveforms of injuries, so that our field of thought can truly be aligned with our being. This is because sound is such a powerful vibration.

This affirmation offers a profound opening for manifestation and healing. Say this affirmation out loud eleven times while inviting your guardian angels to be present. Angels will always come if they are invited, and this beautiful field of thought is where true healing begins.

"There is a light all around me that protects, heals, and nourishes me always."

54

"My breath loves me."

As we receive breath deeply into our lungs, we can feel it nourishing every cell in our body, bringing light, energy, and awareness. If we give ourselves the time to really feel the ongoing inward and outward flow that sustains us, the underlying emotion is trusting that this breath, and the next one and the next one, will be keeping us alive. It is pure love. Our breath loves us so deeply. It will never hurt us. It is always present in us. It started at our birth and will continue our entire life.

In deep gratitude, we can start to understand how God sustains us in the same way. We trust and depend on our breath. We know the next one is coming. Can we believe that God is there for us as well, filling and fulfilling us each and every moment, miracle after miracle? Let us give ourselves the time to stop and feel our breath filling our lungs and circulating throughout our body, with total awe, trust, and gratitude. Let us feel the love each sustaining breath has for us. And may we be like that breath, sustaining and being there in love and perpetual presence for each other as well.

"My breath loves me."

55

"I am free."

How do we let go of our attachment to people or things? We can cut energy cords, write letters full of anger and then burn them, clean out drawers and closets, throw away, recycle, stop spending time with someone, or even spend our energy working SO hard to clear someone from our minds.

I have tried it all. And what I have found is that my only way to freedom is by claiming my truth and loving myself for who I am without worrying what others think. Attachment to things and people drops away by itself when we no longer seek to find ourselves in them. Where can we find ourselves then?

Once we see ourselves as free and love ourselves for our own unique gifts, we no longer need the attachments that trick us into believing they are necessary.

Take a deep breath … exhale … and silently say:

"I am free."

"Today is going to be a great day. I can. I am."

Our first thought each morning creates a vibration that echoes through our day. By choosing an affirmation, a prayer, and a thank you, we create a tone of love that opens the pathway for more goodness in our life and spreads that blessing into the lives of those around us. When our day becomes challenging, that tone keeps on going, keeping us connected to the light of being, holding us in the vibration of the angels, and flowing with the divine wisdom that shines into our hearts.

I love my affirmation first thing the morning, in that delightful moment before getting up, while time seems to stay still. You may find that a gentle reminder is all that is needed to coax our minds into this beautiful habit. So first thing, instead of jumping out of bed, try this affirmation, and see how your day flows. It only takes a moment.

"Today is going to be a great day. I can. I am."

57

"I am guided, protected and loved.
Angels are watching over me always."

Every single day, we can choose to tune in to love and see goodness and joy all around us. Life is wonderfully delicate, exquisite, and far too short to get caught in the grip of fears and worries that our minds can generate. When we trust and surrender to a higher power, we can let go of those fears and experience the reality of the joy surrounding us.

I had a conversation with my sister-in-law before she passed away. Karen's life was very short, and she was especially aware of the beauty on the other side long before she crossed over. It was a cold February afternoon, and as we watched falling snowflakes gently caress the window, I told her how much I love snow. As we looked out, she said, "I know why you love snow, because each snowflake is a small perfect miracle. Each snowflake is an angel. Snow reminds us that we are always with angels. Snow reminds us we are loved. Snow reminds us of the angels who whisper to us with love, and remind us that everything is truly okay."

Karen saw the angels as they were drawing her closer to God. She knew what was happening, and she saw all the beauty instead of the fear.

The miracle in life is to choose love. The more we engage our childhood innocence, the more we can experience joy, yet that innocence continues our entire lives. The more love we share with ourselves and others, the more we attract the most beautiful possibilities.

"I am guided, protected and loved. Angels are watching over me always."

58

"I trust my process."

When an egg cracks open from the outside, it is destroyed. Yet, when an egg cracks open from the inside, there is a rebirth, a new beginning. We must treasure ourselves inside our egg of golden light and love. If we choose to crack open from the inside and honor a new beginning, we reclaim our power first by utilizing the wisdom of the heart. But this is not a time to allow others to take the lead. It is not the time to allow another to hurt us with their own fears. It is a time for us to take the lead and love ourselves so much that even a storm cannot crack us.

But we can choose to crack wide open from the inside outward, with our own power, and with total trust in the divine guidance of timing, with faith, strength and courage. You have everything you need within you. And you have choices. You can open your heart, trusting that God is moving you to open outward when you are ready, and God is showing you how to shift your life into a miracle. Never give up prayers, for prayers have been placed in your heart by God. You are so very loved. And you can choose joy right now.

59

"I AM the mountain."

Old ways of fighting to get ahead are not working anymore. We are seeing through agendas, and our intuitions are empowered with a knowing we almost do not understand.

This mantra teaches us to BE the mountain. Rather than running to find what we are 'missing' or feeling we have to climb mountains to achieve a goal, we can BE the mountain, and let things come to us instead. Rather than looking outside of ourselves, we stay steady and deep within our own radiance.

Each of us has the potential to be strong in our presence and attract miracles into our lives. Every ONE of us. Our very presence is our power when we recognize our potential.

If there are wounds that prevent us from being the beautiful person that we are, then we use all our resources to heal them. It all starts inside. We start with one thought, one positive sense of gratitude, and we can shift the momentum to find ourselves in the flow again.

Take a deep breath and ask your guardian angels to show you the way. BE the mountain. You will attract everything you need to manifest your deepest dreams this way.

Say this mantra for a few minutes every morning and evening:

"I AM the mountain."

"I choose Love. I choose to focus my energy
on the things in life that truly matter."

Our life is precious and miraculous. When we take our last breath, all that really matters is how much we have loved. Yet we worry and become entangled in old belief systems and insecurities, comparing and allowing fear to become prevalent. But we can choose to recognize how fragile and beautiful life is. We can create and nurture a calm, still place inside us, which we can return to again and again to connect with our guiding light.

If we find ourselves becoming entangled in the whirlpools of our lives, we can take a step back into that calm clear center and ask, "At the end of life will this really matter?" And then we can make a shift. Let us not hesitate to create change in action that comes from the space of love. This requires a shift of our momentum, applying the brakes, and choosing to go forward on a path of love.

This is a precious affirmation: "I choose Love. I choose to focus my energy on the things in life that truly matter."

"I steer my life in positive directions by listening to the clear quiet direction of my heart."

This is a mantra for truly stepping into the faith that our hearts are guided by love, and our hearts are guided by God. Let us listen to the quiet voice of our own being and trust our path to the divine within us.

With each new morning, we have a new opportunity for deepening our connection with Grace. With each breath, we can be reminded of the beauty of who we are and trust that God wants the best for us. With each beat of our heart, we can surrender our mind to the wisdom that resides within us. And as we stop, surrender our fear, and listen, we return to our soul and increase our knowing. A miracle-filled life blossoms rapidly from that fertile center.

We all have the same God flowing through each of us, and we are truly connected in each other's hears. As we uplift ourselves, we uplift each other, and as we uplift each other, we uplift ourselves. As we allow intention to clarify, we help all live to their deepest truths as well.

"I steer my life in positive directions by listening to the clear quiet direction of my heart."

62

"With Love all things are possible."

Love is the spark from which creation arises, and with Love all things are possible. All our actions can be distilled down to an underlying momentum sparked by either Love or Fear. When we take actions out of fear, we put up opaque shields that create separation. We do not move forward, and instead shrink back inside our own darkness. We end up like turtles trapped inside our very own shells.

As humans, we have the potential to flow with the grace of the angels. We have so much potential when we simply trust and allow love to work its magic. God flows though us as the light of love. Love attracts more love. Love co-creates. With love we do not need to push through life. With love we just let things come to us by 'being the mountain' and surrendering the need to climb. Life is so much easier when we trust that love is enough, and everything else is flow.

Allow this mantra to help you stay aware of the spark behind your actions. May you trust that love loves you.

63

This is a mantra to affirm our most fundamental miraculous nature. We are vessels of love, and we can recognize the spirit of our loving nature by celebrating the miracles of every moment. Life is full of magical encounters and miraculous transformations.

Can we listen to the still clear voice of our own being? What is our heartfelt desire? What is the most powerful reflection of our loving nature that we can be living into?

"I celebrate the miraculous within me and around me."

"I am following my deepest joy."

When we are in alignment with our happiness, the energy around us becomes radiant, and we attract more things to be happy about. It can be the smallest little moment that creates joy. The key is to take a moment and en-JOY those moments.

When the mind gets caught up in anxiety, fear, or insecurity, we can recognize that it is the mind, then pause. *A Course in Miracles* says a miracle is a shift in perspective from fear to love. The shift is the tricky part. So, pause. Say the affirmation: "I am following my deepest joy." The shift will begin. It is about actually saying it aloud though. Whisper it right now: "I am following my deepest joy." Your brain will begin to agree with you.

Life is too short to allow ourselves to get stuck in the sticky goop. We have things we need to do, but we can choose JOY as we engage in them, even if they are tasks. Having this attitude will change our perspective and transform our doubts into faith. Faith is where the miracles are.

If we are really stuck, we pause and call upon our guardian angels. They will help in an instant. They always do. Even if the miracle does not show up in the way we expect, we are always cared for. All of us.

"I am following my deepest joy."

"I expect miracles to happen."

Great things in life do not appear when we are being pushy and controlling. Magical experiences in life are attracted to us when we visualize and expect the very best outcome, and when we give and serve the highest good of all.

We cannot be afraid to give. We can, however, be thankful for the moments when we forget to give, because those are the moments that teach us the gift of the beauty of giving! Giving to others is the greatest way to increase the field for all possibilities in our own lives.

We all want to live happy, fulfilled, and abundant lives, and there is absolutely nothing wrong with activating our fullest potential and living our lives with victory and magnetism. Actually, we are born to live in joy! But we must first give to others, and expect the best in our own lives as well as the lives of others. There is no room in our world for comparing and competing. Jealousy blocks the miraculous, so shift this way of thinking! If you feel jealous of someone, pray for them, and expect the love to be returned. Observe this. It is like magic.

66

"I accept and approve of myself exactly the way I am."

We are all created as individuals, yet it may seem easier to blend in with the crowd and find ways to fit in with certain groups. But when we do this, we may question ourselves before sharing our deepest vulnerable truths. We can literally wake up in a panic because we are afraid we have said the wrong thing. Our own amazing radiance is hidden, while we feel admiration for others who are courageous enough to be themselves.

The calling of this time is to communicate from our truth. Our truth is what God is asking of us. Truth takes courage. It is time to shine and share the gifts that God gave us, and that shine can only really be true and most magnificent when we share from the full authenticity of who we are. We are learning, growing, and evolving. We shift and we change in beautiful ways, and sometimes that change can seem surprising to others. But, when it comes from our hearts with love and truth, it is almost always beneficial for all. It becomes the missing piece, and that is the enlightenment of the soul.

At each moment of your journey, know that you are beautiful. Trust that God has your hand in perfect synchronicity, and you are beautiful exactly as you are.

67

"Miracles are experienced in the light."

The old paradigm says that people never change. But the truth is that we all have the potential to turn things around. We come unstuck when we make the choice to be unstuck.

It is not good to stay in toxic situations, and the divine love around us reminds us of that daily. When we enable unkind behaviors, we are not serving anyone. But, miracles do exist, and darkness can become light. I have seen transformation, and I have seen people choose to stay stuck. What makes the difference is Love. With love, all things are possible.

We must love ourselves enough for the transformation to occur with the people in our lives. Once we stop allowing people to treat us in inappropriate ways, we give them a chance to get unstuck, and then we are giving them a gift; we are allowing them to create their own miracle by undergoing their own transformation.

We all have the potential for magnificence. Sometimes walking away is the best move because it enables the other person to tap into their magnificence. The key is to do it with love. Miracles happen when love and light are present. If you love someone enough, you can set them free and let them transform into the person they wish to be. If it is meant to be, they will return transformed. This is the miracle.

"Thank you, thank you, thank you."

What better way to start the day? Use this mantra as you state your affirmations, desires, wishes, and dreams. It can be fun to write these things in a card to yourself. Contemplate your hopes and how to find balance while attracting what you desire. The more we express our gratitude, the more we are attracting things into our lives to be grateful for. It is all about the magnitude of resonance, and it is actually quite scientific.

You can also work with this mantra using Child's Pose or Baby Pose. Just sit on your heels, and then bring your heads forward to the ground, almost as if you are bowing. This is the switch. We allow the heart to be higher than the mind, closer to the sky, closer to the angels, and closer to our truth. We allow the mind to support the heart, and take action on earth to support the heart. So many of our seemingly difficult blocks and dramas are created by forgetting to be thankful along the way

Forgiving ourselves is the first step. Surrender is the second. Create a beautiful card for yourself, and put it away in a private place with a gentle prayer and the magical words:

"Thank you, thank you, thank you."

69

"I am a child of Love and Joy.
I am loved and cared for always."

There are so many shifts taking place in our world at this time. The collective consciousness is full of the energies of fear, doubt, frustration, confusion, hurt feelings, sorrow, exhaustion, and loneliness. There are so many opinions outside of our own hearts, it is easy to feel scattered.

Sometimes, we have to go inward and experience the gems that are within us. I grew up with Sunday being the most magical day, our family day. Our father moved to America from Italy in his twenties, and our mother came from England. They met in New York City and had three children, so we were five altogether. We did not have extended family in America until my brother, sister, and I got married.

Throughout our childhood, my father, Giulio, cooked an Italian feast every Sunday. The house always smelled like comfort, and in the winter months, we'd have the fireplace going. Friends would often join us eat Giulio's delicious Sunday creations–he loved to open our home to everyone. He loved to see people smile from his food. He taught us that the greatest pleasure in life was to help others. But he made something else very clear: the importance of alone time early in the morning, time to connect with our inner beings and refuel ourselves.

After my father passed away, I cried on Sundays. Rather than providing my husband and children with an environment of comfort, I found myself feeling sad and longing for my father's amazing energy. My children were babies, and it took a long time for me to snap out of my sorrow. But now we celebrate Sundays again. Do I miss him? Every minute of every day. But now I share my heart on Sundays, in honor of my father, as these are the days I write these meditations.

This mantra reminds us that we have everything we need, even amidst a very busy world, and at times a lonely heart. The angels and God are with us at all times. Repeat this mantra again and again:

I am a child of Love and Joy. I am loved and cared for always.
I am a child of Love and Joy. I am loved and cared for always.
I am a child of Love and Joy. I am loved and cared for always.
I am a child of Love and Joy. I am loved and cared for always.

"Feel the fear, and express love anyway."

Once I was teaching a yoga and prosperity workshop in Costa Rica with Guru Ganesha Singh. To my surprise, he asked me to sing with him on stage at his Kirtan concerts, and I have to say that I found myself incredibly nervous. I love to sing, and I used to sing a lot on stage, even had lead roles in my high school musicals. But over the years, I have not sung much front of others, and I found his invitation both wonderful and incredibly intimidating.

We know, deep inside, when we have to take a step forward, however, and I knew that for my soul I simply had to say yes, feel the fear, and express my love through singing Kirtan anyway. It takes courage to express the love in our soul in the face of our own fear.

We know when we have to take that step onto a new pathway or into a new direction that aligns our actions with our truth. The deepest part of us is pure love, and the deepest calling is when are asked to express love, in any form. Universal love, pure love, without conditions and trusting that God is guiding our hearts. There are myriad excuses that get in the way, and so often we refuse to allow the love and grace of the universe to flow through us. But if we feel our inner fears, hold mindful awareness of all those excuses, and still allow ourselves to be love, express love, and see God in everything, then we make way for rivers of joy to flow through us. It feels wonderful to allow our alignment with our truth to manifest.

That night I sang and sang on that little stage, and it felt like my soul was set free. I felt the sheer joy of singing from the depths of existence radiating into the Grace of the Universe. This mantra reminds us to feel the fear and to love anyway. We can be nervous, we can be full of fear, but if we step into the light and sing our Soul's song, we become liberated from that fear. Feel the fear and love anyway.

71

"Self-acceptance is contagious."

There was a time in my life when I thought I needed to do things outside of myself for there to be action, healing, and forward motion. I learned to write down my goals when I was in college, and then create connections outside of my heart.

But I have learned something, since then.

Goals and external environments mean very little compared to self-acceptance. There is nothing of value outside of ourselves until we completely value who we are. Once we value ourselves, we attract momentum. Once we believe that we are good enough (not perfect), we can move forward with courage. Perfection is an illusion that creates a wall of fear; self-acceptance says: "I am a brat sometimes, but I am human, and I love me for being me." When you accept yourself, your belief becomes contagious.

Please remember to use this mantra as an affirmation. You are affirming it to yourself.

How does it feel?

72

"Healing is happening now,
and the door is open."

This is because there is a force of love that is guiding you, and all the signposts you need will show up when you are ready. It is not a coincidence that you are reading this now. This is Grace. Everything we need is available to us, but we must remove the blocks that hold us back from receiving the magic.

Fear is our biggest obstacle in finding the treasures that life has to offer. How do we move beyond fear? The answers are within. Just set the intention to find healing while tending to your wounds, and then follow the path that is shown from the open door. Take one small step at a time. The hardest part in attracting miracles is the part that we play by closing ourselves off.

Can we agree to stay open, to heal, to grow and to trust? By moving through our fears, and allowing our hearts to be our guides, magic and miracles will flow to us naturally, becoming our reality.

We are living in a very special time, and we are able to co-create miracles every single day of our lives. When we ask for the hand of our angels to guide us, we can trust that we will be guided and shown the way to miracles. Our angels are so very in love with us. They just want us to ask for their assistance.

Ask and ye shall receive.

73

This mantra is another reminder to connect through our hearts, to find beauty amidst all the chaos in the world. Peace is not dependent on what another person does or does not do. It is helpful to remember that no matter what is going on outside ourselves, we can choose peace inside.

The most effective way I have found to practice this lesson is to continue to put my faith in God. There is not a manual for this time of change, but many of us are connecting more and more to higher realms, so that we can bring hope to this struggling world. We are living with a brand-new paradigm, and we have a choice to feel good about ourselves, others and our planet. When we choose love and peace, we receive more love and peace. May we embrace the blessings of our hearts today and always.

"My heart holds my ecstasy."

The angelic realm is of love only, and the angelic realm is up-up-up and of the heart only. We must continue connecting upwards and through our hearts. The mind will only remind us of our insecurities and illusions of separation. The heart holds all the same light rays of the sun. We can shine and regain our power when we live from the radiant expression of the heart.

If we are not invited to the 'party,' we are being called to attend another party–that's all. Connecting upwards reminds us that the party is just an earthly illusion anyway. The truth is that we are all love, and anything else is an illusion created by fear. If it is the fear of another and that is hurting our hearts, we can use the strength of this mantra to release that person from our emotional bond. With love we can let go and trust that if that person remains or is returned in our lives, then that person is meant to be in our lives. Not with fear or attachment, but with trusting that there is a higher road for all.

Allow this mantra to give you the strength to walk away from any situation that has been hurting you. It takes trust and strength which must come from Spirit and our connectivity to the love that comes from the Divine. The physical manifestation of this love, connection, and strength is the HEART.

Repeat this mantra silently for at least three minutes every morning upon waking: "My heart holds my ecstasy."

75

"I let go of the belief that I need approval from anyone other than myself and God."

This is a mantra for releasing what is no longer serving us, including the illusion that we need approval from anyone. We are enough. We are the light of God, ready to shine in our own wonderful and different ways. But we can get caught in insecurities that cause us to seek love and validation from others, and we can build complicated life stories around that need. Then we start living into those stories rather than our own brilliance, and those stories distract us from who we really are.

If we step back and find ourselves going out of the way to live for the approval of others–friends, parents, coworkers, spouses, even people like spiritual teachers–we need to stop and remember the teaching of this mantra.

I can remember seeking approval from my yoga teacher and, in great uncertainty, standing in the teacher's shadow, playing small and obedient. I had nurtured an inner fear that shining brightly would be egotistical, and staying in the shadow of another teacher felt comfortable and safe–until one day I realized that I myself was an artist, and I, too, felt a need to create, and it was hurting me to hide the light that was flowing through me.

It required deep self-investigation and deep daily meditation, some of it quite painful. But this is when I was able to step into neutrality, and let go of the need for approval from anyone except my higher self and God. Letting that need for approval go meant I also released some people in my life who never had my best interest in their heart. Although this was sad, it was liberating. When we release what is no longer serving our highest good, the universe offers us so much more to fill the space.

Since that time, I have received the gift of some truly magical friends who support me tremendously in being a vessel of love. This is the miracle. Once we step into trust, we can expect countless miracles. This was a mantra I created for myself at that time, and still use when I feel myself slipping. I suggest saying it silently to yourself for three minutes when you first wake up in the morning:

"I let go of the belief that I need approval from anyone other than myself and God."

76

"Be not afraid,
but let your world be lit by miracles."
A Course in Miracles

There have been moments in my life where I have felt nearly paralyzed with disappointment. As a child, I believed the world was magical, filled with the most miraculous wonder. But as an adult, my mind became wary of trusting and perceiving things this way. The hurt of feeling betrayed was too painful. The most difficult challenge for me was when a person pretended to be full of love and spirituality, and then privately hurt others. The people who admit to having duality and weaknesses in ego are often souls who make me giggle. The TRUTH sets us free. I would rather be at a party with loud obnoxious people who admit to their flaws, than with people who lecture about spirituality and goodness while talking badly about another in the other room.

One of the greatest bits of wisdom I have learned over the years is to recognize that we can change our minds. No matter what is going on around us, we can change the way we perceive it in our heads. Taking things personally is a waste of precious energy. Fearing what another thinks or says about us prevents us from shining brightly with own our authentic love.

Life is full of challenges. The key is to stay present in the field of love no matter what is going on around us. How do we do this? By trusting that nothing real can be threatened.

Staying authentic with ourselves allows us to walk with Grace. Remember that God is the Love within us. When we choose love, life becomes blissful. We feel ease when we can acknowledge that we are surrounded by our own protective vibration of love. Where love is absent, fear becomes prevalent. A true miracle is a shift in consciousness from fear to love. By training our minds to recognize that nothing authentic can be threatened, and anything that is not made of love is merely an illusion, this is the avenue for peace.

Love is reality. Fear is illusion.

"Be not afraid, but let your world be lit by miracles."

"My reality is love, my lesson is love, and I am learning more about love in every moment."

This mantra tells us that every moment teaches us, informs us, and guides us where we need go inside ourselves to find the soft human connection of love, caring, and consideration. That is true success. We can choose to learn, or we can choose to chase after our mind – that's our choice, always.

The world is changing so fast, and we are feeling challenged on a daily basis to keep up with the pace. Our bodies have spent millions of years evolving to thrive in a non-electrical, non-digital, non-mechanized world. Suddenly we have smart phones, texts, social media, and a completely new set of rules. Everyone is struggling to adapt. Even newspapers go out of business in a virtual world. It can feel so confusing. Everything is new, and it seems impossible to detect what is natural and what is virtual. It's so easy to get hurt. But the one reality remains the same through all time. In the evolution of our soul, we ultimately learn that the one thing that is at our core is still there, shining, patiently and joyously. The most important lesson is that our interpersonal connections, the love we share, the moments of mutual uplifting energy, are what is real. We gain wisdom from our interconnectivity, and we can share this with others so the vibration of the world can be uplifted.

"My reality is love, my lesson is love, I am taught more about love in every moment."

"I am determined to see things differently."

Stay steady with these words and observe how they protect your inner soul: "I am determined to see things differently."

Free yourself in knowing that you can change the way you see the world. If what you see is not bringing you joy, change your perception. Focus on something that makes you smile, and choose that thought in place of the old pattern. As we heal our mind by releasing unhealed thoughts, we begin to see a road of beautiful flowers, and our peace is reflected back into the world we see.

79

"The Love in my Heart protects me."

Love is the most potent protective force of the Universe. The connective force of love becomes the protective force as well, just like the force of gravity holding atoms together. When we recognize the highest truth in each other and within ourselves, at the highest frequency of surrender to the Divine, then with our attention we are creating a force that is so incredibly strong, so incredibly bonded, that we may stand tall though all changes and challenges.

Love brings like frequencies together in an astonishing way that amplifies and solidifies so we become many times stronger than we are as individuals. With the connective force of love, our consciousness becomes a fortress that can withstand the crashing waves of emotions, the pulls of this lifetime, and all of the greed, egos, and trials of the world. Our love energy holds us together in its purity and proves that light overtakes the darkness, and beauty prevails. This is our lesson:

"The Love in my Heart protects me."

"In my grace is my power."

Now more than ever, we need to learn how live in grace with each other. We can do this by allowing God to work miracles rather than struggling for personal gain. When we relax and allow the abundance of the Universe to fill our hearts with compassion, then our source shifts from feeling limited to feeling part of infinite Grace. In nature, everything flows in harmony, creating rivers, flowers, stars, galaxies, and babies. Every one of us is part of this flow, and we are all part of the grace of God. But most of us have been brought up in a culture that supports competition, comparison, and rivalry. When we start comparing ourselves to others and competing for what is actually infinite abundance, it creates a separation at the very root of our beings.

The reality is that we are One with all there is, and we can choose to vibrate and communicate on a wavelength of Love. When we love each other, we love ourselves. Loving ourselves, we love each other. Helping one, we help all. I firmly believe this is our natural way. It is not something to work for, but something to relax and surrender into. We must allow ourselves to re-align with the divine flow of Grace that is with us all the time. We can find more energy, more strength, and more wisdom when we become one with the divine flow that breathes into us, giving us life.

Remember this is not about being a doormat, it is about being bold and strong enough to be powerful human beings. We must learn to speak our truth, to fight for what we believe in, to reclaim our own individual power, and to do it all with GRACE. We are being called to let our light shine brightly without fear. Our life lessons remind us that when whenever we react out of fear or anger, we actually lose our strength. When we take a breath and speak from our hearts, we reclaim our strength in our grace.

"In my Grace is my power."

"Miracles Are Real"

Once I was on a conference call with Oprah and the amazing Belief team, and we were asked to write #beliefin3words. I wrote "Miracles Are Real," and in that moment, I felt the miraculous beauty of a dream coming true for me: I was a guest at the United Nations for a screening of Oprah's new series.

I am sharing this with you because I truly believe God loves us all so much, and supports our dreams. My dream is to share my love with the world in an authentic and healing way so that my presence can inspire others to trust that a higher realm exists, and that through the power of our own energy, we can attract our heart's desires.

Being part of this incredible Belief team has expanded my heart in profound ways, and I truly believe we are all longing to know that we have an impact on the world in one way or another.

When Oprah was talking at the United Nations. I felt as though I was listening to a friend chatting about life. She talked about how she knew for sure that we were ALL the same—all of us are longing for connection and approval. She also discussed divine timing and how things play out in unexpected and magnificent ways when we listen in stillness.

During the reception after the screening, I gently touched Oprah's arm, and again it felt like I was touching a dear friend.

Oprah has inspired me so much as a vessel of divine love. Her mission is to show the world a better way, and her words are demonstrative of the sacred beauty of HOPE and BELIEF.

"Miracles are REAL."

And YOU are entitled to receive your miracle. All you have to do is BELIEVE.

82

*"I am not alone in experiencing
the effects of my seeing."
A Course in Miracles*

This mantra reminds us that the thoughts which give rise to what we see are never neutral or unimportant. This mantra reminds us that our minds are joined. It refers to how we see things, our perceptions. I know for myself that when I allow my thoughts to come from fear, the illusion of doubt is easily antagonized. Yet, while sitting in stillness and plugging my heart into the Divine, I am able to recognize that love prevails.

What do we long for more than anything else? Connection to one another. What do we fear more than anything else? Separation. Quieting the mind with deep breathing and trust, we see that we are never alone. Use this mantra to identify your own perceptions, and observe that we are all connected by a thin thread.

We are divinely interwoven. The most beautiful math equation is YOU + ME = ONE. Can you elevate your own thoughts in order to elevate another?

This lesson needs application for just one minute a day. Give it a try:

"I am not alone in experiencing the effects of my seeing."

83

"I release and let go.
I allow God to move in my soul."

Whenever I let go of my fear and follow the inner guidance of my heart, miracles happen without any effort, like the gentle blossoming of a flower. On the other hand, whenever I hold tightly to patterns that don't serve my highest good, because I am afraid to give up control, I end up repeating patterns that take me one step forward and two steps back.

Is it possible that you are reading this right now because you are being asked by Spirit to be courageous? Can you trust that your inner guidance is real and Divine and in everyone's highest good? If you listen to your heart, you will hear the sweet song of permission. God is not only giving you permission, but calling you, ever so patiently.

The time is NOW. You are being called to use your senses to see and hear all the reminders that God is giving you permission to start your new chapter. Just reading this is lovely, but the miracles happen when we shift our brain chemistry and believe the truth we know in our hearts:

"I release and I let go. I allow God to move in my soul."

"Divine Beloved, change me into someone who can give with complete ease and abundance, knowing You are the unlimited Source of All."
~ Tosha Silver

Tosha Silver's words are so powerful: "Let me be an easy open conduit for Your prosperity. Let me trust that all of my own needs are always met in amazing ways and it is safe to give freely as my heart guides me. And equally, please change me into someone who can feel wildly open to receiving. Let me know my own value, beauty, and worthiness without question. Let me allow others the supreme pleasure of giving to me. Let me feel worthy to receive in every possible way. And let me extend kindness to all who need, feeling compassion and understanding in even the hardest situations. Change me into One who can fully love, forgive and accept myself, so I may carry your Light without restriction. Let everything that needs to go, go. Let everything that needs to come, come. I am utterly your own. You are Me. I am You. We are One. All is well."

This mantra is a beautiful prayer for change and transformation. If you feel drawn, let it enter your Being, releasing any old ideas of constriction or limitation, and reviving your true essence as expansive radiant Light.

"As long as I believe that anger brings me something I really want, I will be in conflict, and peace will elude me."
A Course in Miracles

Sometimes we are not even conscious of why we feel angry. Most of the time, the resentments appear due to childhood wounds that we have repressed, but we blame outside circumstances. Anger is an uncomfortable emotion. We do not like ourselves when we are snippy. It is not our true nature. How do we shift out of anger?

1. We recognize that expressing ourselves is healthy, yet we also remember that harboring and holding anger patterns never brings us peace and happiness. In fact, anger lowers our frequency and therefore keeps love away.

2. We cannot experience love and anger (a form of fear) at the same time, so we must throw the anger in the garbage. Delete it like you would delete an old email–the trash can on the computer is magical. The words just dissolve.

3. We remind ourselves that we can love others into new patterns and habits. We can't force them to change, but we can use love as a tool to help them grow. It takes patience, but it is so worth the conscious effort.

4. Gratitude. Sit with gratitude. In the beginning you may feel angry and frustrated as the distractions of life pause when

we quiet in our minds. The key is to stay steady and observe. Allow the thoughts of gratitude to miraculously melt away the anger.

5. Trust that there is always hope, no matter how things appear. We can use compassion to lead us forward. Force just brings us out of sync, but flow aligns us with love. Have compassion for where people are. Pray for them rather than judging them. Chances are they are in pain, and your love can miraculously heal something in their hearts.

6. Spend time with the people who lift you up.

7. Stay with this lesson. Apply it daily for five minutes, and use the energy of the collective consciousness to find the natural state of being in your heart, which is JOY.

Remind yourself of this truth: Miracles occur naturally when LOVE is present.

86

"If we could learn to live from the level of the soul, we would see that the best most luminous parts of ourselves are connected to all the rhythms of the universe.
We would truly know ourselves as the miracle-makers we are capable of being."

Spiritual teachings that intimidate others are not true spiritual teachings. Honesty, Integrity, and Divinity are essential for living our lives to our fullest potential. The universe has its very own intelligence, and we attract what we are grateful for with ease when we release the walls of illusion and truly walk our talk.

The world is responsive to our desires when we take risks based on integrity and honesty. We are human. We are not perfect, but we are doing our best. On a soul level, we hold awareness that we are part of an abundant world, but on a human level our negative minds are always working to protect our hearts. We must practice moving out of our egos and dropping into our heart space. Sometimes we are more angelic than others, yet while we live here on Earth, we are human.

Happiness requires honesty. If we are going to uplift others, we need to be real, and that includes sharing our humanity. We are sharing our vulnerabilities one at a time and helping one another along the way. This is true spirituality. And with this formula, we can truly love ourselves and then love and support others:

"I attract my deepest desires when I allow the walls of illusion and fear to dissolve into truth and Love."

> "I am sustained by Love. I am sustained by Love. I am sustained by Love."

This is a lesson to release old paradigm of separation. With these five simple words, we move out of a state of yearning and into the mindset of peace, wholeness and contentment.

"I am sustained by LOVE."

Undoing old belief systems in our subconscious minds creates space for us to activate the light within our hearts. You are light unto yourself, which spreads out to others. We cannot underestimate our potential anymore. It is too painful to hide the gifts that Spirit has given each and every one of us.

Meditate on these words for at least five minutes every day. If we say them and mean them, we will not just understand them intellectually; we will leave behind insecurities, and we will alter our relationships with everything. I am ready for this one. Are you? GO!

"Everything is in perfect divine order."

Sometimes, it is hard for us to understand how everything can be in 'perfect divine order' when things seem to be going wrong, or when loved ones pass away. But no matter what happens, we need to remember that the universe has a divine intelligence, and the love around us will always sustain us. No matter what is going on in our lives, if we can see each moment as a gift, we can learn to laugh again.

How is it perfect order when you lose a loved one? It is perfect order because they become closer to us than ever before. When we lose a loved one, we gain an angel. When we change our perceptions to the miraculous, everything changes color. Darkness becomes Light again. With Light, we attract more Light. With Light, we attract more Love.

Experiment with this miracle mantra by repeating it silently to yourself for three minutes:

"Everything is in perfect divine order."

"Today I choose neither to judge nor interpret anyone's motives or behavior."
A Course in Miracles

This is a challenging lesson on so many levels. But it will help you conserve precious life energy.

Some people do really awful things. There is illness of the mind in our world. The news can make us cry, and the behaviors of others can be shocking. But it is not healthy for us to sit and ponder over the intentions or motives of others. Our brains are biased. These minds of ours will tell us we did something to deserve it, or we did nothing to deserve it.

The mind will play games with us. But we don't need to know why anyone else acts out in strange or hurtful ways; we only need to learn to let it go. We waste energy trying to understand. We take things personally. We allow ourselves to become victims. Can we stop this behavior in ourselves? Can we continue to love and shine our light even on those who have hurt us?

God's plan works. So let's surrender. Trust that what comes around goes around. When we feel separate from others, it is often because we are judging. When someone changes the script we have written for them, we feel conflicted and hurt. What can we do? Shift our perception. Free ourselves by giving up the illusion that we have control. Give our concerns to a higher force. When we feel triggered, rejected, or confused, let's practice releasing the mind games.

Shift thoughts of fear to love by saying 'delete' out loud to anything that triggers a negative emotion. Say 'yes' to joy and happiness. Remember there is a higher force with you at all times. Whatever you are going through now may be a blessing to prepare you for a miracle. Choose Love. Choose Light. Breathe. Breathe deeply.

LOVE is patient.

"The Divine permeates all things."

The work of this mantra is to meditate on our trust in the universal flow of Grace. We think we need to take action and manipulate our circumstances. Our mind teases us into thinking we need to play the game. Yet, the Divine permeates EVERYTHING! So what can we do, when we feel the need to intervene? We can lift our vibration by recognizing that we are deserving of a beautiful life. We can close our eyes with gratitude and say "thank you" to God for the many blessings around us at all times. The infinite potential for love, abundance, and miracles comes from opening our hearts and staying in the flow.

Speaking words of goodness while taking actions aligned with love and gratitude can cause an immediate increase in our vibration. Science is proving that sound vibrations alone can move objects. Imagine what love and faith can attract!

"The Divine permeates all things." God's plan works. Our own individual plans allow for disappointments. Can we put our energy and work into trusting the divine map and elevating our frequencies with love, hope, and gratitude? Our heartfelt LOVE can increase the energy fields around everything.

Why do we allow the fear? Because we are human, and we need to do our work with faith. Today, choose love. We are in this together. We are One.

91

"Infinite patience produces immediate effects."
A Course in Miracles

Sometimes, stillness is the best thing to do. Sometimes it is the solution to a problem. When in doubt, we stay with our breath and contain our reactions. Words can be very hurtful when perceived the wrong way.

So practice patience. Have patience with yourself and patience with others. Have patience with the Universe. Trust in the ebb and flow of our world. Our dreams and desires manifest so much faster when we are patient. Pushing and controlling can make us feel more productive, but the universe responds to the light in our energy fields. The more we can be patient and surrender to the flow, the faster our dreams will be impacted positively. Absolute patience is the same as loving acceptance. Loving acceptance with positive intentions and relaxation can bring things into being. What is our deepest desire? Can we align with it, and then surrender it with patience? Can we trust?

*"I release all the drama, and
I receive energy from peace and simplicity."*

This is a message of surrender. We are all moving so fast. The energy around us is accelerated as well. Science tells us that energy waves are the substance of the universe. Every thought we think and every action we take has a direct effect on someone and something else. Our practice is to bring positive energy to others, and in turn, spend time in nature to release any heavy energy we may have absorbed.

Energy is directly influenced by our actions, words, and THOUGHTS. Our actions, words, and thoughts produce our feeling state. Our feeling state becomes a currency which can purchase gifts of simplicity, healing, happiness, and peace.

This mantra can help you focus your energy on small, simple, and manageable steps to move into a life of miracles. Simplicity is a form of abundance. Surrender and peace are forms of perfect health. Sitting and closing our eyes in meditation is one of the greatest gifts we can give ourselves right now.

"I release all the drama, and I receive energy from peace and simplicity."

"Peace to my mind. Let all my thoughts be still."

Sometimes I feel as though my thoughts are robbing my soul of the richness in life. My insecurities and fears seem to have more power over my heart wisdom, until I stop and recognize the game my mind is playing in the moment. We cannot allow the mind to win. It is full of old wounds. That is why we love children so much–their purity is all heart-based. Can we become children ourselves this week? Let's go for it. Quiet the thoughts that rob you of your bliss. Your heart space can win, and that is the true path to love and abundance.

A world without fear would be a world full of Love. We can have this now, in our own lives. So, shhh … May your mind be still. Shhh, may your heart be open.

Love awaits you.

94

"Within me is deep Peace."

In the core of our being is a reservoir of complete stillness. It remains there, contentedly, while we rush around in the business of our lives, making plans upon plans. We spend our days planning our next move and crossing things off our list, only to add new things and new plans, and soon it becomes very easy not to notice that inner space anymore.

Nonetheless, our inner reservoir of peace remains strong and still, because it is holding our essence. It can never go away, but can only be concealed. We can practice finding it again by stopping the incessant plans and constant mental projection into the future, and instead giving ourselves a moment, a minute, or a morning, simply saying, "I am enough, I am enough right now, and within me is deep Peace."

We re-discover our inner reservoir of peace by breathing deeply into it, enjoying the feel of our lungs filling with air. We listen, we smell, we taste the essence of the moment, and we allow it in, touching our inner being. If we practice regularly, breathing in to the inner reservoir of peace, it becomes more and more apparent. Waking up and remembering to be mindful of our breath works wonders.

Take a moment right now to stop planning and find the peace within.

95

> "As I change my mind, I change my life, remind-
> ing me that no matter what the problem,
> love is the answer."

I find so much comfort in this mantra. It is a good one to work with as soon as you wake up. Our thoughts are so powerful, and we can change them at our free will. When we change our mindset, we are changing our experiences as well. At any moment, we can choose peace over conflict and love over fear. Just take a deep breath.

There is so much freedom when we change our perception. When we seek love instead of faults, we teach others how to do the same. We can contain ourselves. We can shift our perceptions with some quiet time, and then even amidst the external energy of others, we can choose love.

This lesson saves me from feeling overwhelmingly compelled to fight for what I believe. It guides me to use the power of love and hope to manifest a magic wand, and this saves precious life force energy, while keeping us safe from the attack of another. See how it works for you.

"I can look upon everything I experience today
as a positive lesson."

This mantra tends to be something that we resist tremendously. How can something that hurts so deeply be a 'positive' in our lives? Many of the negative experiences in the world seem to have absolutely NO positive aspects. Yet, it is possible to learn, to grow, and to find opportunities from the experiences that bring disappointment or sorrow. That is what we can control: how we PERCEIVE the benefits or anguish from the experience.

Some of the most beautiful pieces of art were created from people who felt so deeply. Music is the same. We learn lessons and we grow when we are put into uncomfortable situations that we long to move out of. The opportunity comes when we LISTEN to the callings of our souls.

My father passed away in the most awful way. His funeral was the saddest day of my life, because I experienced another loss while we were saying goodbye to him. I felt like I wouldn't make it that day. It was anguish with a capital A. But I grew so much. The sadness still arrives at times, but now I have an understanding and a calling to help others in an entirely new way.

Every experience offers a positive lesson from which we can learn and generate more love, acceptance, compassion, tolerance, and forgiveness. Say this mantra for five minutes at a time to shift your mindset:

"I can look upon everything I experience today as a positive lesson."

"Today I will choose to no longer see any value in comparing myself with others."

When we compare ourselves to others, we are being unloving to our own souls. Aspiring to learn qualities from people we admire is a beautiful thing. But judging oneself in comparison to another takes away from our precious life force. The ocean is vast and abundant. There is so much beauty in the world to go around. Sharing our uniqueness and truth with others, while appreciating their gifts as well, is a quality that truly enhances our lives. We don't always know what another person may be going through in their lives anyhow.

Comparison hurts. Love heals. The more we uplift and assist others, the more happiness we are attracting into our own lives. We find joy in the joy of another when we love ourselves deeply, and we listen to the call of our souls. Let us align ourselves with harmony, now.

"I am enough."

This is a powerful mantra. We are all blessed by the same light shining inside. There is no lack and no shortfall. So often we feel we have to live up to external standards. We can fall into patterns of running from inadequacy or constantly feeling a need to prove something. Sometimes we search for an external definition of success. The truth is that our success is in our awareness. Trusting that we are always held in the lap of a loving universe is a true form of fulfillment.

Yes, there is always more to do. It is too easy for us these days with all this technology to fear that we are missing out on something if we sit in our stillness. Yet, the truth is that our stillness is the attracting force to all forms of abundance. With this mantra, take a step back, breathe, and allow yourself to be amazed by your own existence.

"I am enough" is a mantra of your own value on a soul level. You are not inadequate. You are so beautiful. There is perfection this very moment. Can you go about your day while remembering this, and being kind and loving to yourself? You are enough. You are bountiful. You are loved for who you are. You are embraced in the light of love. Always.

"Safety always returns."

Our world can feel like a very unsafe place these days. But there are so many beautiful angels whispering to us. They say, "Shhh! It is all okay."

When I was in college, one of my favorite professors shared something with me that I will remember forever. She expressed that her greatest memories were of moments when she was going through something. Those were the moments when she grew the most. When life ebbs and flows, she said, rather than thinking God is doing something *to* us, recognize that God is actually doing something *for* us.

You are safe. You are safer when you follow your heart and take a leap of faith because living a life without moving towards fulfilling your destiny is painful. Being stuck is so much more difficult than taking steps, even the steps that feel frightening.

Can we trust that there is a plethora of angels smiling upon us and whispering,

"If we knew what we know now when we were in your shoes, we would have always known how safe we were. Why wait?"

Our own inner state is where true safety resides. If we have a roof over our heads, food to eat and LOVE as fuel, there is no need to find safety anywhere else. We have everything we need.

No one can protect us from our minds, and our lives reflect our inner state. So we do our practice together. One day at a time. We change our minds, and recognize that fear is just fear. It is not real. Love is here for us, all the time.

"Safety always returns."

100

"I release my attachment to taking things personally."

The world is shifting, and many people are experiencing super sensitivity to subtle energies, often with dramatically increased feelings of empathy and interconnection with others. Super sensitivity takes a lot of getting used to. This mantra helps us to release the old paradigm of feeling that we ourselves are the object of these sensations. We are being called to understand our center, to know the difference between what is within and what is without. This can be so confusing. It is as though we can feel others' actions almost as if they were our own. We can start to feel responsible for others' lives. This is the remains of the old way, the lingering survival mechanism that allowed humans to take action in the face of discomfort. But we do not control what others do, and even though we may now feel them as part of us, what they do is not about us. It is about them.

We must learn to adjust our reactions, like toddlers learning to walk. We can feel others' lives in full loving awareness, and we can lend a hand, pray, love, serve, and be deeply involved in our circle with all of our heart and soul, while also maintaining the neutral awareness of Grace flowing through each of us equally. What others do is not about us personally. It is about where they are in the midst of their own process—their own soul, their own karma, their own lessons, their own handicaps, and their own genius.

There is no question that we have all been very hurt by the actions of others. But if we go beyond the discomfort, beyond thinking it is about us, beyond self-blame, beyond anger, we may see an opportunity for growth. Remember, it is never about us when we are hurt. It is always about the one who is hurting. So how can we respond? We interact, we love, we heal in our amazing capacity to be vessels of the divine, uplifting Earth. But we have to give up the old feeling that we are at the center of everything that happens. God is in the center. We have to give up the feeling that we are victims. Spirit has gifted us all with our own power. When we see the divine spirit flowing through everyone, then we can also start to know who we are in the midst of it. Is it simple? No. But it is essential for our own sense of peace at this time of spiritual evolution. We are all experiencing stronger sensitivities these days. You are never alone.

101

"I am one with life. I am one with now."

Use this mantra to reflect on the concept of connection. Being one with life helps us to see the bigger picture. We are eternal spiritual beings that are having a human experience with brains on fire! These minds of ours are full of *bjkpplkhgtyukhbhuxozzzzo*. That is not a typo. It is symbolic of the state of confusion our subconscious minds blurt out. One way to get out of this fear-based mindset is to live in the present moment with your breath. Can you allow life to be the dancer, and you to be the dance?

Making peace with the present moment is being one with all that is. Recognize that we are never alone. We are always supported and loved. We are worthy. We are invited to the biggest party, the one with all the dancing of the heart, the party where the angels sing. We don't need to think about living life, we can allow life to live for us.

Flow. The field that permeates all things is made of energy and love. This field is the dance of life. Dance in a field of flowers today (even if only in your mind!), and become one with all that is.

"I am one with life. I am one with now."

102

"I am allowing for all possibilities."

This mantra is a gentle reminder to allow for all possibilities. So often we hold back on what we envision as possible. When we put limits on our vibration with thoughts like, oh, that is impossible, or there is no chance, then we are preventing possibilities from manifesting.

These times are calling for faith. In this sacred season of transformation, renewal, rebirth, and miracles, we can call on the innocence of our hearts to guide our way into a miraculous future. We can use the power of "I AM" as a mantra to renew and grow into our conscious envisioning. The shared wisdom of all religious traditions calls us to transform, to believe, and to trust. Trust is the realm of the heart. Don't hold back on what you envision. Don't let the mind get in the way. Believe, trust, and take a step into the light, and the beauty of your own potential.

Say this mantra in the morning and before you go to sleep to create a magical shift by letting it steep into your subconscious mind:

"I am allowing for all possibilities."

"Truth unites. Truth never separates."

Sometimes I think we need a support group for us deep feelers. I am not sure why some people have a capacity to let things go, while others feel everything on such a deep level. Sometimes I cry for the pain in the world, or even the pain of people I do not know, or on seeing the discomfort of an animal in pain. Thankfully, Spirit has blessed many sensitive souls with the capacity to know that there is a palace of light and perfection which we can touch upon by closing our eyes with deep breathing and alignment with Source.

Use this affirmation to uplift and bring peace into your mind, body, and soul. Emotions can be on the rise, and deep feelers will benefit from allowing the tears to flow. If you feel like the odd one, just remember that many of us feel this way! This is an opportune time to confront your fears and be courageous in staying true to your heart's deepest desires.

We are all vulnerable, and some of us feel things with greater sensitivity. Some of us protect, and some of us have incredible coping mechanisms to eliminate discomfort. Yet we are all going through huge changes together, and it is in joining with our true hearts that the world can become a more joyful place. "Truth unites. Truth never separates." Who we are is who we are meant to be. Fitting into a box of 'acceptance' never truly feeds the soul. But by listening to our own unique voice, we can experience growth and expansion. This is a brilliant and fertile time. Can we unite and accept one another for who we are?

"Truth unites. Truth never separates." Connection comes from within, because first we must connect with our own hearts. From there we can share and love and connect with others in a natural and truthful way. Be open to receive the benefits of this mantra:

"Truth unites. Truth never separates."

"I rise above thought and experience the pure joy of my heart."

True happiness is something we discover within us. It is the joy that resides in the core of our beings. Happiness is temporary if we seek and find it anywhere else. We can spend forever searching this way and that, trying to find happiness in wealth, love, entertainment, clothes, even missions and moments. These are all beautiful gifts, but true joy is perpetual, flowing like a timeless stream of light through our hearts when we transcend the neurotic thoughts of the mind and become aware of our inner energy in the moment.

Our minds can fall into a habitual pattern of creating thousands of negative reasons why joy is not appropriate. To free ourselves from this pattern, we must consciously practice enjoying at a soul level, softening and allowing our natural inner beauty to permeate our cells. And then, amazingly, the pattern starts to shift. We change our brain chemistry to one of enjoyment, and this affirmation can help:

"I rise above thought and experience the pure joy of my heart."

105

"I am truth."

This mantra teaches us to trust the flow of inner knowing as it permeates through our entire mind, body, and soul. We must have faith in our gut instincts. Our intuitions are so much stronger than our mind games.

One of my favorite stories from Hans Christian Anderson is *The Emperor's New Clothes*. In this story, two weavers promise the emperor a new suit of clothes that is invisible to those who are unfit for their positions. The emperor parades around naked, yet all the adults are ashamed thinking they just can't see the beautiful cloth. It is a child who is courageous and speaks out: "He isn't wearing any clothes!"

We are conditioned to stay in our neutral minds and keep quiet. Often, we do not trust the pangs of inner knowings. We do not speak out when others do not see what we see. I am finding that Spirit speaks to my heart. It does not even matter how 'ridiculous' my knowings may seem. I have learned to trust them. It is not easy for me to see through so much these days. It has even been painful at times. But I truly believe there is a purpose for it. There is a reason our intuitions are speaking loudly at this time. Our world is changing very quickly.

Please trust that you know so much more than you 'think' you know. When in doubt, sit with your eyes closed and repeat:

"I am truth. I am truth. I am truth."

"I take time for self-love and reflection."

This affirmation is a reminder to work with the rhythms and cycles of life, to flow and glow like the moon in all its phases.

If you are feeling more tired than usual, you might be receiving a sign to slow down. So drink more water, eat whole unprocessed foods, spend time in nature, laugh, rest, spend time with close friends and family who love you exactly as you are, write in your journal, take a walk, make a gratitude list, or simply sit and know you are enough in your stillness.

Stating the "I" in a mantra is a great way to remind ourselves that we are worthy of loving ourselves. It is not an egotistical statement, it is simply a statement of nurture. We deserve to nourish ourselves.

Sending light from my heart to yours as I sit in my stillness and see you in yours.

107

"I believe. I believe. I believe."

Always follow the path of your heart. This is where the miracles are activated. It is the home of your deepest calling, one step at a time.

Be careful to step only on the stones that light your soul. The darker stones are there only to trick the thief of the mind. They are detours, always with lessons, but we are ready to move beyond making the same mistakes. The heart knows sweetness and Grace, so follow the Song that vibrates in your deepest knowing.

When our desires are aligned with the highest good of all, there is a Divine support system that is activated. There is enough for All. Lack is an illusion. You have everything you need inside of your heart, so let it shine. Be courageous. Leave disbelief behind and onto the path of least resistance. There is nothing to fear.

"I believe. I believe. I believe."

108

As we embrace this time we see that everything in our lives is here to bless us. And how can fear live in us if we have forgiven ourselves? Embrace this beautiful day! From the mouth of my young son, "Choose love"

"There is nothing to fear."

109

"I am the light flowing though my heart."

There is a special light that gives us our energy. We are the grace flowing through the physical. And that light is always striving to merge with its own vast love. A gateway is open right now, illuminated, with angels all around, waiting and ready to be stepped into. It is the gateway to our own truth, and we need courage to move forward.

The light of God is so tangible right now. The veil has become thin, and we feel the touch, asking us to move, to trust, and to allow the blessings of the angels. It can feel quite unsettling. We must trust that God is with us. Divine infinite grace is guiding our hearts, right there with us every step, to make good choices. We surrender, we bow, we allow, we practice our meditation, we practice our faith, and we trust the hand of God in our lives.

This affirmation will help you identify as the divine light that flows through our heart. Try saying it three times each morning and night:

"I am the light flowing through my heart, I am the light flowing through my heart, I am the light flowing though my heart."

110

"Love is power."

With this mantra, we are activating a heightened brain frequency. Our minds may be over-thinking, but now is the time to awaken and clear any old, stagnant thoughts that are rooted in our subconscious minds. This mantra can help bring clarity and cleansing to the chatter, so we can follow our bliss. The heart holds the wisdom.

It is love's power that can move mountains. Human beings searching for control and power seem to have forgotten this simple truth. Manipulation and fear-based chatter do not have force. Love is power. Love is power. Love is power.

If the ego screams at this, allow it for a moment, then say shhh. We know better than to listen to that voice. The heart whispers the path of health, wealth, and happiness. When we give to another, we are giving to ourselves. If we want something, the best way to manifest it is by giving it to someone else first. It doesn't mean we allow others to use us as doormats! It means that with love, we have a power way beyond anyone else's fear-based agenda.

"Love is power."

We can give our love, and if we don't receive it back from where we are hoping to get it, we know that it is not our loss. It will arrive in perfect timing as part of the Divine Plan from a means way beyond our imaginations.

111

"I am love. I rest in the light of this truth.
I am enough. I am free to be me."

This is a mantra for trusting our intuition and knowing when to strive and when to rest. Can we find balance in the doing and being? Let's not get caught up in manifesting. Instead let's go inside our hearts and trust. Just trust that the love vibration will attract all that we need. We are expressions of love and compassion. Love is everywhere. It is in the air we are breathing at this moment. Breathe deeply. Have faith. Follow your heart.

This is a simple but powerful message. Let's raise our Love vibration together!

"I am LOVE. I rest in the light of this truth."

Acknowledgements

Words do not seem to be enough to express the love, gratitude and warmth I hold in my heart for so many of you reading this.

I'll do my best to put my heart into words as I let the love flow through my fingers.

First, I'd like to mention that this book was born in the quiet moments of early morning breath, stillness and listening. Throughout a span of three years, these affirmations were created one week at a time on Sunday mornings when the noise of the world softened enough for love to speak.

Gabriella and Christian, thank you so much for giving mommy that space and time to meditate and write. You always seemed to know when I was in my quiet zone, and somehow you both understood that you were in that energy field with me. The field of love and the place the angels dance is a deep part of your understanding too. I thank God for your love of the angelic realm. I love you both more than words can say.

Charles, twenty six years ago when we hardly knew one another, you asked my father for my hand in marriage, in his strong Italian accent he said: "Yes, as long as you always care for Karena. She is very sensitive."

Thank you for trusting what our souls knew. Soulmates are real. Thank you for always caring for deep feelings. You are my rock. You are my sunshine. You are my protector and I am not afraid to admit that you help me to stay feminine, child-like and gentle. I loved you the moment I met you, because I recognized you. Thank God for that day. I love you so much.

To my beautiful mother, Mama Beryl: Thank you for your courage to take that ship from England to America on your own when you were at such a tender, young and vulnerable age. Thank you for delivering babies into this world and teaching us all about midwifery and holistic medicine. Your courage to stand up to others has helped me find my voice. Thank you from the bottom of my heart for having patience with me when I was a child who struggled to fit into this world. And thank you for showing us respect and service for humanity, for teaching your children to give back and to choose love again and again. I am so grateful that God gave you a second chance at life. You are my mommy forever, and the love I feel for you is eternal.

To daddy: I have never stopped missing you. Thank you for knowing me, seeing me, loving me and always celebrating me. I treasured every single moment on this earth with you. Your glow and radiance filled this world, and it's a miracle that you overcame such a hard life growing up in Italy to become the father you were. Somehow your knowing of starvation and abuse transformed your trauma into giving and love. You were the most generous man that many of us who knew you had ever met. Your light continues to shine in so many hearts and homes. You were a rare gem on earth, and you are a treasure in heaven. I will see you again on the other side, but as you know, I have much work to do here first. I love you, Giulio Ferrari.

To my big brother, Robert and my little sister, Stephanie: I love you both so very much. When either of you hurt, my heart hurts too. I will always and forever be your Kinsky. I am so thankful to mom and dad for giving me the best gifts they ever gave me- both of you. You are both such amazing gifts to this world, too.

Thank you to all the second mothers in my life. Growing up with grandparents and extended family members living overseas creates an intimacy between the friends we cherish. I'm so grateful for mothers, and especially the ones who have mothered me. To nana, thank you for your love and consistency. Thank you for always listening so beautifully. Thank you for spending those precious moments with Gabriella and Christian while they were growing up. You are truly a blessing. To Sue and Nancy, thank you both for your all American motherly love. I am forever grateful for your homes and your huge nurturing heart. Thank you for loving the Ferrari family the way you have for all these years. We love you too.

To my nieces and nephews: you know how much your auntie Kina loves you. I hope you read this book to your babies one day, and that they and you all remember the love that created you. And to Michael, who left us too early to be with his mom on the other side, we know you are a free eagle soaring through the sky now. I miss you, I forgive you and I love you so much.

In this moment, I offer my deepest gratitude to the angels in the unseen realms of light who so faithfully guide and protect us. Thank you for the gentle whispers, the subtle nudges, and the moments of grace that arrive exactly when they are need-ed. Again and again, you remind us that we are held, loved, and never truly alone. Thank you. Thank you. Thank you.

To the sacred presence of the Divine that breathes through all things: Oh how I love you. Thank you for the endless well of compassion, presence, unconditional love and miraculous mo-ments that make healing possible. These affirmations are small reflections of that infinite love.

I am deeply and forever grateful to the teachers, healers, students, clients, kindred souls and very special friends (you know who you are and I love you from the depths of my heart!) who have walked beside me on this journey. Your wisdom, encouragement and open hearts have been bright lanterns along the path of life and the frightening road less traveled. Thank you, Sally, for persuading me to publish the affirmations into a book. Thank you, Kate, for assisting me in formatting each of the miracle mantras from weekly Facebook posts into a book format. Thank you, Sarah, for being such a wonderful assistant to me all these years.

Thank you, Maile, for being such an honest and detail oriented editor who helped me make this book possible.

To Bruce Springsteen, who always helped me to see and know that I was not the only different one. Thank you for always being supportive and for constantly sharing your kindness with Gabriella and Christian. Your wise words are your authentic care for this world have truly helped me to feel less alone when the world looked so different for a while.

To those who have shared their stories, their wounds, and their courage to heal, thank you. Your vulnerability is a sacred offering, and your journeys have inspired many of the prayers and affirmations within these pages.

And finally, to you, dear reader. If these words have found their way into your hands, trust that it is not by accident. May these affirmations feel like gentle wings of light around your heart, reminding you that you are guided, protected and so profoundly loved.

As the veil between heaven and earth thins more and more everyday, may it be the norm to speak of Love.

May angels continue to guide us, protect us and join our hearts as we do our part in bringing light to this world.

May everything flow in perfect and divine timing and may peace prevail on earth as it does in heaven.

May God bless us always.

With my love, devotion and gratitude,

Karena xo

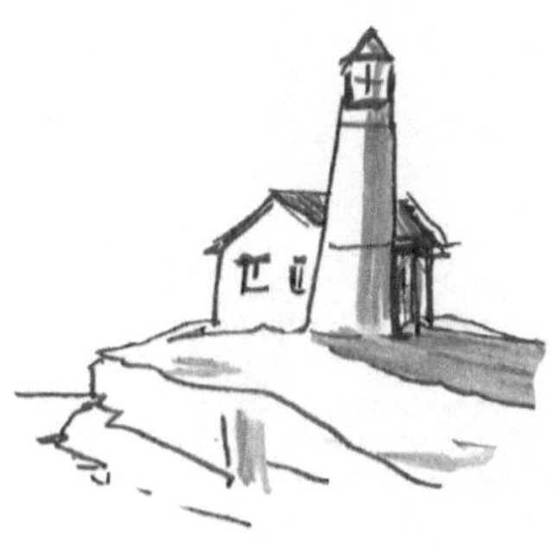

WINTER ISLAND PRESS
SALEM, MASSACHUSETTS

Winter Island Press edits and publishes books that reflect the breadth and bounty of human experience. Our roster of authors represents a vibrant tapestry of voices. We are delighted to work with both seasoned writers and promising debut authors who contribute to the literary mosaic that defines Winter Island Press. We value creativity, originality, and craftsmanship. From fun and potent fiction to thought-provoking nonfiction and poetry, Winter Island Press publications offer narratives that leave a lasting impact on readers' hearts and minds.

If you have a compelling manuscript that aligns with our vision, or even a great idea for one, we'd love to hear from you. Connect with us through our website, winterislandpress.com.